Teaching Interactive Skills in Health Care

Ann Faulkner

SRN, RCNT, MA, MLitt, DipEd, PhD

Professor of Communication Studies in Health Care
The Medical School
University of Sheffield

and

Deputy Director
Trent Palliative Care Centre
Sheffield

CHAPMAN & HALL
London · Glasgow · New York · Tokyo · Melbourne · Madras

Published by Chapman & Hall, 2–6 Boundary Row, London SE1 8HN

Chapman & Hall, 2–6 Boundary Row, London SE1 8HN, UK

Blackie Academic & Professional, Wester Cleddens Road, Bishopbriggs, Glasgow G64 2NZ, UK

Chapman & Hall Inc., 29 West 35th Street, New York NY10001, USA

Chapman & Hall Japan, Thomson Publishing Japan, Hirakawacho Nemoto Building, 6F, 1-7-11 Hirakawa-cho, Chiyoda-ku, Tokyo 102, Japan

Chapman & Hall Australia, Thomas Nelson Australia, 102 Dodds Street, South Melbourne, Victoria 3205, Australia

Chapman & Hall India, R. Seshadri, 32 Second Main Road, CIT East, Madras 600 035, India

Distributed in the USA and Canada by Singular Publishing Group Inc., 4284 41st Street, San Diego, California 92105
First edition 1993

© 1993 Ann Faulkner

Typeset in 10/12pt Palatino by EXPO Holdings, Malaysia
Printed in Great Britain by Page Bros, Norwich

ISBN 0 412 45870 5   1 56593 227 7 (USA)

A catalogue record for this book is available from the British Library

Library of Congress Cataloging-in-Publication data available

∞ Printed on permanent acid-free text paper, manufactured in accordance with the proposed ANSI/NISO Z 39.48-199X and ANSI Z 39.48-1984

Teaching Interactive Skills in Health Care

This book is for Mary – for the sunshine she brought with her, and her constant reminder of the importance of a balance between work and play.

Contents

Preface   viii
Acknowledgements   ix

PART ONE: Teaching Strategies for Interactive Skills

     1 Safety in learning   3

     2 The formal/semi-formal setting   15

     3 Using video-taped material   23

     4 Role play   34

     5 The use of audio feedback   49

     6 The discussion session   63

PART TWO: Problems, Costs and Measurement

     7 Potential difficulties   77

     8 Handling the cost of caring   88

     9 Evaluation   97

PART THREE: Learning from Research

     10 The need to teach effective interaction   109
        strategies

     11 The skills of communication   117

     12 A model for teaching   126

     Appendix: Resources

        Further reading   134

        Video-tapes   135

Index   137

Preface

I have been involved in teaching teachers for a considerable number of years. First, in teaching methods, in general, for nurses on the MSc course in the Department of Nursing in Manchester (when it was also possible to gain a teaching qualification). This was followed by teaching interactive methods particularly suited to helping individuals to improve their ability to interact effectively with patients and families in health care.

It has been rewarding to carry out research in this area for this has given insights into methods that are effective, and those which still require development and further evaluation. This does not relegate the informal evaluation from health professionals which has helped considerably in my own learning process.

My work was much enhanced by the period of time when Dr Peter Maguire and I refined and developed our skills and mounted both basic and teaching courses for health professionals who wished to run workshops in their own locality. Due to changing work commitments, Peter has had to withdraw from these courses, which are supported by Help the Hospices and continue twice each year for doctors, nurses and other health professionals.

This book is written in an attempt to share some of my experience of using teaching methods with those who wish to develop their own skills in teaching effective communication in health care. I have relied heavily on my own experiences to illustrate the text and, once again, in writing about this area, make no apologies for my pragmatic approach.

I hope that some of my enthusiasm will transmit itself to the readers of this book and that some day communication as a subject will find itself in its true place, in the curricula of all health care professionals.

Ann Faulkner
Sheffield

Acknowledgements

There are many to thank without whom this book would not have been possible. Organizations such as the (then) Health Education Council, the Cancer Research Campaign, and Help the Hospices all funded research and/or teaching initiatives which have helped develop knowledge, skills and strategies. I learned much from working with colleagues equally committed to improving communication in health care, and much of that learning is, I hope, encapsulated within this book.

My family and friends have been ever supportive, both in understanding the time I required to write, and in their ability to help me maintain a sense of balance.

Finally, but very importantly, I would like to thank Barbara Grimbley for typing the manuscript and for her patience throughout the whole endeavour.

PART ONE

Teaching Strategies for Interactive Skills

CHAPTER ONE

Safety in learning

There is no doubt that teaching interactive skills is more demanding on both the tutor and the student than teaching factual material. The variety of teaching methods all put some demand on the students and indeed the tutor to participate and take risks. There is, of course, a place for the factual lecture, though even this may be broken down and facilitated rather than simply presented with the expectation that participants will listen and absorb the information. Indeed, throughout the teaching of interactive skills, when quite a lot of time is required to practise in a relatively safe environment, one of the decisions that has to be made is in terms of how much factual material should be given.

It is argued here that only those theories that are mutually related to the learning in hand are necessary as part of the course. Other theories of communication, counselling and interaction in health care can be covered by background reading. This helps the students to take responsibility for part of their own learning and bring back to the classroom thoughts and questions about particular issues.

DEMANDS ON THE TUTOR

Student set agenda

If the student is going to improve and build on skills based on a contextualized programme that has been devised by the group (see Chapter 12), the tutor or tutors will have to be prepared to teach very much 'on the hoof'. Inevitably, this will occasionally mean that tutors are faced with a situation with which they themselves may not be familiar. Owning this will increase the student's respect for the tutor because implicit in the fact that nobody knows it all is also the fact that what is taught is taught by someone who has the experience and knowledge to do so. This level of honesty, although sometimes painful, will also encourage the students to admit when they themselves need help with a particular situation.

Student reactions

Using experiential teaching methods also means that students are more likely, because they become involved, to have problems within the learning experience. This demands that the tutor is able to screen for signs of distress, agitation or other signs that someone is upset by what is going on. The ability to take swift, decisive action, sometimes to protect the participant, sometimes to protect the group, requires a high level of concentration on the part of the tutor. Similarly, dealing with hostility and non-participation (Chapter 8) may make considerable demands on the tutor who is trying to give attention to the whole group.

Finding positives

In order to facilitate learning while helping participants to feel safe and valued, positive feedback is a very effective teaching tool. This can be very demanding, particularly at the beginning of the course or workshop where students are (1) finding their way and (2) often making considerable errors in the way in which they interact with patients.

In real or simulated situations, the maxim that there is always something positive to say about any situation looks very good on paper, but in fact can be quite difficult to achieve. Experience and careful observation of each situation can make this task more manageable, and tutors can improve this skill dramatically over time. The effect on the participant of positive feedback which builds on whatever skills they have brought with them can be very rewarding, whereas a critical approach to performance can damage student/teacher relationships.

It can be seen that teaching interactive skills may be demanding in a way that straight lecturing seldom is. It requires the ability to think on your feet, to be big enough to say, 'I'm sorry, I can't help with that problem', to pick up problems in the group sooner rather than later, and to avoid negative comment as far as possible. It is draining but endlessly exciting work.

DEMANDS ON STUDENTS

Participation

Students who are used to lectures as a means of learning can be very threatened by experiential methods. In a lecture a student is free to listen or to let his or her mind run free; they may take notes or they may indeed write home to mother during the lecture depending on how keen they are to gain knowledge, and sometimes how keen they are to have the relevant material to pass their exams.

With experiential teaching methods it is very difficult for the student to be uninvolved; in a relatively small group where the student is expected to participate, non-participation will be noticed by both the tutor and other group members. What is, however, most threatening appears to be the problem of putting ones skills on the line in front of colleagues and sometimes friends. This is particularly true when the group is comprised of trained and often senior people.

Threat of experiential methods

It will be seen in Chapter 4, on role play, that this is perhaps the most threatening teaching method of all for the student. Many participants in a group may have already had worrying experiences of this form of learning. The tutor, therefore, cannot assume that the students will feel safe in interactive learning.

Safety

The tutor/facilitator will need to reassure participants that the situations in which they find themselves, during the course of a workshop, will be made as safe as is possible for them. No-one can promise absolute safety because no tutor knows exactly what 'luggage' the student has brought with them. It will be seen later in this chapter that various psychological situations can be reawakened in experiential learning, and although this is relatively rare it has to be addressed.

The student may also be fearful that they will somehow be made to look silly or that they will somehow not measure up to other members of the group. If, for example, participants are meeting for the first time as part of a group for a workshop, they may well look around and feel somehow that other people in the group must know more than they do or be more clever than they are.

TUTOR'S RESPONSIBILITIES

The group

For these reasons the tutor has a responsibility to give time, thought and effort to setting up the group at the beginning of the course or workshop. This may be easier if the group being taught has already met before as perhaps part of a more general course in which teaching effective interactive skills is just one part. However, this cannot be assumed because often one is more concerned at looking silly in front of friends than in front of relative strangers. One strategy that is very helpful is to point out that everybody is in the same boat and that the teaching methods to be employed will apply to everybody.

Similarly with a group that is new to each other, particularly if that group is multidisciplinary and contains, for example, doctors, nurses, social workers and others. What has to be addressed here is the barriers that may exist between, for example, doctors and nurses. The tutor can make it explicit at the beginning of the course or workshop that for the purposes of the teaching everybody will be seen to be a participant who wants to improve their skills, and barriers just seem to disappear. In an early mixed workshop it was amusing to hear a nurse say to a doctor, 'Do you know, I think I could begin to believe that doctors are human beings with problems too!'

(a)   Size

It has been demonstrated that experiential methods require considerable concentration on the part of the tutor. Size of group is a considerable factor in maintaining a safe learning environment, for the larger the group the less able is the tutor to monitor the whole group and its reactions to the situation currently in hand. If there is one tutor only teaching the material, then the group should be no larger than eight to 12, 12 being an absolute maximum. If there are two tutors available as in the Help the Hospices workshops (Maguire and Faulkner, 1988), then group size can increase to a maximum of 16 to 20. This large group would be split into smaller groups for role play and other sessions as appropriate.

A group can be too small, though there are a variety of beliefs about this. Six is probably the most comfortable small group in terms of minimum number. Anything less and the people within the group are under considerable pressure.

It would be very difficult to run a role play session with only four participants since two would be taking the part of patient and health professional and two would be observers. They would be constantly changing and constantly under pressure, either to enact a particular scenario or to be able to generate ideas on the way forward.

Others would argue that the smaller the group the more intensive the teaching. The counter-argument to that is that the smaller the group the shorter the time before that group is totally drained and needing to be lifted to something much lighter.

Overall, the problems with size are usually that the group is much larger than is reasonable if experiential methods are to be used. This can certainly pose problems in colleges of nursing where a tutor may be responsible for a group of 40 or more. What is then required is negotiation for splitting the group with a colleague. For example, a tutor teaching interactive skills would take half the group while the other half might have a library session or another practical session where a smaller group is preferable. This does require covering the same material twice but it is a feasible way to teach effectively even with large groups. Problems may arise in organization of a timetable if colleagues are unsympathetic to the problems, but, with patience, *quid pro quos* are usually possible.

(b) Group cohesion

If a group has not worked together before, some time needs to be spent on building group cohesion. Only then will participants trust each other enough to disclose their fears and worries about the course and the problems that they personally have brought to the course to do with their work and improving their skills.

Exercises

In early workshops run with Gaynor Nurse (unpublished) exercises were used in dyads and triads. Typically, participants would be paired and each have five minutes to tell the other something about themselves. The large group would then reform and each participant would introduce the other one in their own pair. These sorts of exercises can help participants to get to know a few people in the first part of a course or workshop. A very good book by Brandes and Philips (1978) gives a whole variety of exercises to help a group to warm up and to gel. In multidisciplinary workshops (Maguire and Faulkner, 1988) these exercises tended to irritate health professionals who felt that they were adult enough to get on with the work.

These exercises should not be dismissed since they certainly have value in some situations. The risk is that they tend to have a party flavour to them; for example, an exercise where each person has a name of an animal pinned onto their back, and, by questioning other members of the group, have to find out who they are. The purpose of the exercise is clear, that is, to help people to talk to strangers and to get to know them, but this purpose is often obscured by the luggage that the participants have brought with them, that is, the need to learn and improve their skills in time that is precious and has been given up from normal duties.

Relevant tasks

What has been found to be effective on two levels is the agenda-setting tasks described in Chapter 12, for not only does it help to identify the areas that are required to be covered in the workshop, it also helps people to begin to talk to each other about an area that is of common interest. Without exception, at the end of the agenda-setting exercise, part of the group is beginning to know each other very well and this leads on to the sharing between the two groups that engenders further building of trust and relationships.

One exercise from the Brandes and Philips book which seems to be particularly successful with student nurses or medical students is a variation of S7 – 'Fear in a Hat'. The exercise goes as follows:

> Tutor: 'Most of us bring some worries to a new situation – what it will be like, what it will demand of you – and so I want to start this course by asking you to write down your major worry about the course and then put it into this box that I'm going to bring round, so can you all find a small piece of paper?'

Usually there is a bit of scrabbling round for paper but everybody writes something and some people take longer than others, but when a few individuals appear to have written something, the exercise proceeds as follows:

> Tutor: 'Can you screw up your piece of paper because I'm coming round now to collect them. Those of you that haven't quite finished, don't worry I'll come round again.'

After all the pieces have been collected the tutor shakes them up and again talks to the group:

> Tutor: 'Well, you've all hopefully got rid of a worry but what I want you to do now is to take a worry out of the box when I bring it round. If you can see obviously which is your own worry, please don't take that one out again. When you've got your new worry, I want you to look at it, think about it and then when everybody has got a new worry I'm going to ask them to say just a sentence about it to try and sum up how they might feel about it if it did belong to them.'

The strength of this game is that the worries are often fairly common. Several individuals may have the same worry. For example, they are concerned about the prospect of doing role play. Others may be concerned about being made to look silly, and as each person looks at the worry and says a word about it there is often a great deal of empathizing as follows:

> Tutor: Jean, can you tell me which worry you've picked out?
> Jean: Yes, this person says that they are very worried that they won't be able to come up to the standard of everybody else.
> Tutor: Can you say something about that worry Jean?
> Jean: Well, I suppose I want to say, 'Join the club' because that's worrying me too.

Often too this particular game brings some humour early on into the workshop. One example was of a small workshop where people were going to work together intensively for two or three days well away from a city centre. No less than three participants had written down that their main worry was that they would not be able to get to the bank during opening hours. In that instance the tutor was able to reassure them that indeed they would get an adequate break for shopping and other things to give them much needed space during their intensive workshop.

In summary, the exercises that help a group to gel are those that they can 'buy into' without feeling in any way diminished. Sharing of common problems, as in the agenda-setting exercise, or sharing worries tend to make the group gel because suddenly they find that they are not the only one with this or that worry, or feeling a little less than perfect. This allows the individuals to begin to feel part of a group that will work together as equals all with strengths and weaknesses.

WORKING WITH THE GROUP

Every group is different in the teaching situation in terms of what the members bring with them, what they require from the teacher, and what they make of new ideas and concepts given them. There are, however, two distinctly different types of group.

Captive audience

The captive audience describes a group who are there because they *have* to be there. This applies to most teaching programmes for nurses and medical students and other health care workers where learning to interact effectively is part of the curriculum. Participants do not have a great deal of choice as to whether or not to attend in such a situation, and learning in this type of group will take place where the students are highly motivated primarily by the tutor.

Self-selection

The second type of group comprises those who are there because they are highly motivated. This applies particularly to workshops, seminars and courses where there is no obligation to come but participants can choose to attend in order to improve their skills. In this instance the tutor has to maintain and encourage the motivation that the students have brought with them.

INTRODUCTIONS

In spite of the above, no assumptions should be made as to why a participant is within a group, or about what they require from the workshop or course that they are currently attending. For this reason it is useful to include a question about why you are here in the introductions. The start of a course or a workshop might include introductions as follows:

Tutor: I'd like to start by telling you something about me and why I think I have a right to be here and work with you on how to improve the way that you interact with patients and families in your care. After that, I'd like each of you to say who you are so that I can have an idea of where you come from and what you do. I'd also like to know, in a sentence, why you chose to come to this workshop, or if coming wasn't your idea but someone else's.

It will soon become apparent if individuals are on the course or workshop because they want to be there or whether indeed there is some other reason. It may be, for example, that someone has been sent on a workshop because it was felt necessary for them to be there. They may not say in their introduction that they have been sent but there is usually some sort of indication that shows that the individual is not very happy. The following is an example:

Participant: I'm Mary Smith. I'm a staff nurse at St Always Hospice.
Tutor: Can you tell us why you are on this course?
Mary: To learn more about communication skills, I suppose.

Tutor: It doesn't sound as if you are too happy to be here.
Mary: Well, it was my nursing officer. She suggested that I might do well to come.
Tutor: And you?
Mary: Well, I had to cancel my holiday.
Tutor: I'm sorry about that Mary. Let's hope we can make it worth your while to be here.

In the above exchange the nurse was making it clear that her wishes had not been considered when the decision to send her on the course was made. It is important to know this because it can foretell difficulties for that staff nurse if she is particularly resentful, and this can have an effect on the whole group. In situations like this it is often worthwhile to have a private word with the participant at a coffee or lunch break to check the level of discontent at being on a course that has disrupted her personal life.

These introductions are the beginning of sharing between the group; the people who come because they have aspirations to improve the way they work with their patients; those who come because somebody else thought it was a good idea; and those who are there as part of their development that has been negotiated with senior staff where they work. If warm-up exercises follow straight on from introductions then the group is very likely to gel and come back from their first coffee break ready to share their ideas and work on the programme that is agreed.

PLANNING THE PROGRAMME

The programme may be planned well in advance of the teaching or, as suggested in Chapter 12, it may be planned as a result of agenda-setting exercises on the parts of the participants. In either event, thought will need to be given to the particular methods to be used, the order in which they are used and the safety of the participants in terms of what they are expected to give to the group. The teaching method used will be based on the material to be taught. For example, it is well known that someone acting the part of a depressed person in role play can themselves begin to feel very low. For this reason, if teaching about depression, role play would not seem to be the most suitable teaching method.

SELECTION OF METHOD

In making learning as safe as possible for the participants then the material taught should move from the simple to the complex and the methods used should move from the safest to the least safe. From this it will be seen that no workshop or course on communication skills would start with role play, nor yet would such a course start with a session that was seen to be particularly heavy or draining, such as bereavement.

In terms of method, a lecture or a facilitated group discussion can be a very safe way to start the work of the course and, indeed, it will be seen from future chapters that this first session can lay down the ground rules for the workshop and ensure that everyone is using the same language in terms of what is meant by skills, knowledge and attitudes to effective communication.

In planning the remaining programme, methods should be used to suit the material to be covered, to move the group on, in as safe a way as possible, and to give a mix to participants to prevent 'sameness' which can lead to participants becoming restless.

Time	Day 1	Day 2	Day 3
9.15 9.30	Introduction – setting the scene Identifying problems	Assessment II (discussion) 10.15 Safety rules for role play	Working with children (video session)
10.30	Coffee	Coffee	Coffee
11.00	Agenda setting Prioritizing areas of concern	Role play 1. Assessment 2. Denial	Role play 1. Anger 2. Collusion
12.30	Lunch	Lunch	Lunch
1.45	Negotiating programme 1. The language of communication	Role play 1. Breaking bad news 2. Answering difficult questions	Unfinished business (discussion) to include hope/spiritual issues 2.45 Support/survival
3.45	Tea	Tea	Tea
4.15 –5.45	Assessment 1 (video session)	Advocacy/confrontation (video session)	Evaluation Close 5.45 pm

Figure 1.1 Example of programme for a three-day workshop.

1.	Breaking bad news
2.	Collusion
3.	Answering difficult questions
4.	Assessment
5.	Hope – how to give when outlook poor
6.	Working with children when a parent is dying
7.	Denial/unrealistic expectations
8.	Confrontation/advocacy
9.	Spiritual issues
10.	Dealing with anger

Figure 1.2   Typical top 10 agenda items for workshop.

It is also important to plan the programme so that sessions end on a positive or light note. In a workshop, for example, the session at the end of each day should be selected to cover a topic which is not too heavy. It may be that role play sessions, for example, may finish at the tea-break and that a video with some humour may be discussed in the final session. Figure 1.1 shows a programme for a three-day workshop for doctors, nurses and social workers. It will be seen that the material covered relates to the agenda agreed by a group (Figure 1.2) but was arranged in such a way to end each day on a manageable level, and leave the last day arranged so that participants left on a positive note.

SUMMARY

In this chapter it has been seen that using experiential methods for teaching effective interaction with patients and their families requires effort from both tutors and participants in terms of risks and disclosure. It has also been seen that the methods used – for example, discussion, video demonstration, role play and audio feedback – can be used in such a way to take the participant from the relatively safe interactive learning to the relatively risky. It is the tutor's responsibility to ensure that each situation is as safe as is possible.

The size of group has been considered as a very important matter when planning experiential learning; also, that the group will work best if there is time given to setting up group cohesion, whether by warm-up exercises, agenda-setting exercises or other means that are both effective for a particular group and accepted by them as reasonable. It has also been seen that there is a relationship between the material to be taught and the most appropriate method of teaching it. In the following chapters, methods will be considered so that tutors can choose what is most appropriate for the material to be covered.

REFERENCES

Brandes, D. and Philips, H. (1978) *The Gamester's Handbook*, Hutchinson, London.
Maguire, P. and Faulkner, A. (1988) How to improve the counselling skills of doctors and nurses in cancer care. *British Medical Journal*, **297**, 847–9.

CHAPTER TWO

The formal/semi-formal session

Although a course or workshop can be taught largely using experiential methods, it is very useful to have a formal/semi-formal session at the beginning to set the scene for what will come later, to give information about what the course does or does not aim to do, for setting parameters on the sort of material which can be covered, and for identifying a common language in terms of what is meant by effective interaction, in relation to skills, attitudes and knowledge bases.

SCENE SETTING

In scene setting, it is worth negotiating with the group what will be covered in the course or workshop, how it will be covered, the methods to be used and what will be expected from the group. Even if the agenda has been set by the group, they will wish to know the weight to be given to particular areas of need and the teaching methods that are to be used.

By negotiating in this way participants will have the opportunity to raise any questions and concerns so that everyone has a clear idea of what is going to happen in the time available. This open and honest approach avoids participants being anxious about things that might be sprung on them unexpectedly and with which they might find difficulty in dealing. It also gives the opportunity for negotiation and agreement on areas of genuine concern.

EXPERTISE WITHIN THE GROUP

If the group is multidisciplinary, it is obvious that there will be very different levels of expertise within that group. This may seem daunting to the tutor/s who may wonder how there are going to be common learning sessions when there are wide variations in knowledge, attitudes and skills. In fact, these differing levels of expertise can be very useful in a group that is working well together, for it allows a considerable amount of sharing. It also allows the tutor to fully exploit her role as facilitator rather than having to be seen as the fount of all knowledge. What is important is to make it clear to the group that the expertise is acknowledged and accepted. For example:

> 'The aim of this course/workshop is to build on the skills and ex-pertise that you have each brought with you. We recognize that there is a good deal of knowledge and experience within the room which we are hoping to use, so that at the end of the course/workshop you will all feel that you have enhanced and developed your own ex-pertise. We hope you will then practise in the clinical situation and come back to us at follow-up and tell us what has worked for you and whether new issues have been raised as a result. We also need to know what hasn't worked for you so that we can look again at the area in perhaps more depth or from a different perspective.'

In this way, each participant will feel valued for what they have person-ally brought to the course and this can help to avoid feelings of being 'de-skilled' when teaching starts.

Similarly, it is important to acknowledge that individuals have come to the course/workshop because they know themselves that they need to improve their interaction with patients, relatives and, indeed, their colleagues. This again can be done in a positive way, particularly when talking about what will be required in terms of role play or, if it is to be used, audio feedback. This will be discussed in the relevant chapters but it is worth acknowledging at the beginning of the course/workshop that individuals are on the course because they recognize that they have deficiencies and that this in turn means that they will occasionally get stuck, be unable to answer questions or have immediate answers to problems that are raised in teaching sessions.

SETTING PARAMETERS

There is often a good deal of concern within a group as to what the teaching is going to be all about. This is as true of a group of medical students, nursing students or, indeed, a multidisciplinary group of trained staff. This concern may be exacerbated if the word 'counselling' is in the title of the course or workshop. It is therefore quite important before any formal teaching starts to give clear ideas of what the course is all about. For example, the British Association of Counselling makes a clear distinction between counselling skills, which are pertinent to all health professionals, and counselling, which is a therapeutic relationship entered into by a counsellor who is fully trained in the relevant skills.

In defining the aims of the course/workshop in this way, participants will be comforted to know that they are not going to be expected to take on a therapeutic role as a fully fledged counsellor, but that they are, hopefully, going to improve their skills. This means that they will learn to properly assess their patients and, as a result, make sure that care is based on what the patients' real problems are rather than what their supposed problems are. This, coupled with the participants' input to the agenda, will have a strong motivating effect since everything that subsequently happens will be tied to clinical reality rather than theoretical issues that may not seem relevant to the particular participant.

It is also important to make clear that there is no element of competition in the teaching. Since each participant will have brought their own particular level of skills, knowledge and attitudes to effective communication, what they take away will also be highly individual and it is worth pointing out to participants that the only person that any of them are in competition with is themselves. This again can ease tensions, particularly in multidisciplinary workshops where staff nurses, for example, may feel that somehow they have to measure up to medical colleagues. This is an imagined rather than a real risk, as has been shown in the work of Maguire and Faulkner (Faulkner, 1992) where baseline skills of doctors, nurses and other health care workers show very little difference between the grades or professions.

NEGOTIATING PARTICIPATION

It cannot be assumed that because individuals are within a group to learn to improve their interaction with patients' families and colleagues, that they will wish to participate. This is particularly true of the captive group of students, whether they be nurses, doctors or other health care professionals. In fact, in working with medical students it has been found that they are very surprised if they come into a module where they are expected to do more than take notes in response to formal lectures. As a result it is worthwhile to negotiate participation based on the benefits that can be seen to accrue for the participants.

Negotiating participation can best be done when describing the different teaching methods that will be used. For example, identifying a common language could certainly be done by a straight lecture in which the participants simply take notes. The tutor might point this out to the group as an initial chance for them to think about participating. This might be approached as follows:

'We're shortly going on to talk about identifying a common language. This means that we will all be sure right from the beginning that we are talking about the same things and that we have, hopefully, the same beliefs about the knowledge, attitudes and skills required for effective interaction. I could give you that as a straight lecture with a hand-out, but I thought it might help the group to get to know each other a bit better and certainly set the scene for the sort of interaction I am hoping for if we do this by discussion.

'In other words, I will facilitate the session and work on what you can each give to the discussion so that we can sort out what we mean by effective communication. Is anybody unhappy with that idea? No. I want you to tell me if you are unhappy because I believe we will work best together if we are open and honest with each other. What we will be doing is pooling the expertise that is in the room and I will come in only when there seems to be a gap. Please do not feel worried if you do not know all the answers. If you did, you would not need to be here.'

The tutor would then map out the different teaching methods that will be used and the amount of participation that will be involved. For example, if everybody has been asked to bring an audio tape (see Chapter 5), then it will be negotiated that everybody will have a chance to play part of their tape for feedback and positive comment.

If the teaching is for a short period where everybody cannot take part, then there may be more problems than would be expected if everyone can be involved. If only a few people can be involved than it can give everybody the chance to opt out unless a clear contract is agreed. This will be further considered in Chapters 4 and 5.

PLANNING A SESSION ON 'COMMON LANGUAGE'

The planning for a formal session is very important, especially if a considerable amount of input is expected from participants. The planning needs to include the objectives of the session, how they are to be met, and how the available time is to be allotted. If time is limited, choices may have to be made between encouraging group participation and ensuring that all objectives are met.

Objectives

In a session on the common language of interaction, the first objectives may be to identify the key skills of effective communication (Chapter 11) and give examples of their use within an assessment interview. Further objectives may, if time permits, be to put these skills into perspective with non-verbal behaviour, knowledge and attitudes required. It is helpful if the tutor makes an *aide memoir* of the material to be covered, in note form. This is crucial if participants are to be encouraged to generate the material, for the tutor will be able to see at a glance which items have not been identified. This will allow tutor input when participants' contributions have been exhausted.

Meeting objectives

If the session includes group participation, questions may be pre-planned to encourage participation. Initially these questions may need to be very specific in order to generate offers from the group. Consider the following two questions:

1. 'We are talking today about a common language of effective interaction. Who is going to make a start?'
2. 'We are talking today about a common language of effective interaction which includes some key skills. I'd like you to think of particular skills and I will put them up. Can someone start us off?'

Question 1 is too vague and may generate equally vague answers. Question 2 is focused and therefore helps the participants to react in an equally focused way.

In addition to formulating some key questions in advance, it is also useful to make a note of relevant examples to be used in the event of the group being unable to offer examples of their own to illustrate skills. This gives the tutor assurance that he/she can deal with any 'gaps' in the interaction, and underline material offered if necessary.

Since material is unlikely to be offered in logical order, it is also useful to plan a summary of the session in advance which can be put up on a flip chart or produced as a hand-out.

Allotting time

When objectives have been set, and the format of the session has been planned, it is useful to go through the material and give an actual time to each part of the session. This has several functions:

1. It highlights whether there is too much, or too little, material for the session;
2. It encourages discipline in teaching;
3. It encourages the notion of giving proportional time to the various areas to be covered;
4. It can aid thinking in terms of optimum time for sessions which will help with future negotiation and planning for different areas of the course/workshop.

THE SESSION

The overall aim of a session on 'common' language is to identify the skills required for effective interaction. If this session involves participants, the tutor will encourage participation if he/she can accept all offers in a positive way. Each item should be written up on a flip chart

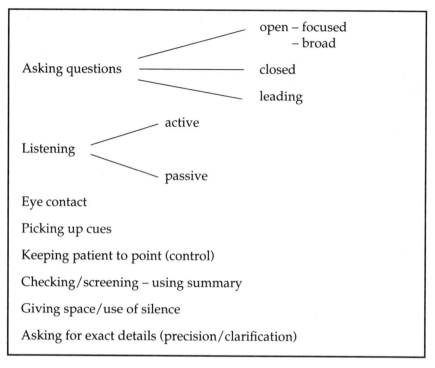

Figure 2.1   List of skills of communication generated by workshop.

before the individual is asked to say a little more about the particular item. For example, the first thing offered under a heading of 'Skills' on the flip chart might be 'Asking questions'. The tutor, hoping to tease out the different type of questions – such as open, closed and leading – will ask participants what sort of questions there are. Normally there is someone within the group who can describe an open question, someone who can describe a closed question and perhaps also say something about leading questions.

This means that in the first few minutes of the session, several people have contributed and the tutor will be able to build a picture on the flip chart starting with questioning and filling in other skills as they are given. Figure 2.1 shows a typical list of skills which are not in any order of merit, but which have been extracted from the group along with examples and also with differentiations as in 'Asking questions'.

Inevitably some skills will be missed and the tutor, after screening for the missing ones, may offer one of the missing skills and ask if any member of the group can talk about it. The interaction might go as follows:

Tutor: 'Well, we've certainly got most of the skills up on the board
            now. Is anyone able to give me any others?'
            (Pause)

	'Well, one that we haven't got up there is 'clarification'. Can anyone in the group tell me what we mean by 'clarification'?'
Sally:	'Yes, I remember this one now – it's to do with being sure that we're clear on what the patient really means.'
Tutor:	'Why is that important, Sally?'
Sally:	'Well, I suppose if we're not clear we could make mistakes.'
Tutor:	'Yes, and it's often tied to the fact that there's lot of ambiguity in our language. We use many words that can have different meanings, like 'normal'. A lovely example is of the man who was asked if he ate a normal breakfast and he replied that, yes of course he did, but I'm sure you can all see that what's normal for one person may be quite different for someone else. How many of you would say you ate a normal breakfast? I'll guess that what you do have for breakfast will be anything from a cup of coffee on the hoof right through to eggs and bacon, toast and goodness knows what.' (Laughter.)

If there is time, the above can be even better illustrated by actually asking members of the group what they eat for breakfast, and checking out to everyone's amusement the very different beliefs people have about what is a normal diet. These examples are often remembered far better than a straight explanation of clarification.

Attitudes and knowledge can also be dealt with in the same way when identifying a common language. The group between them will often have a very clear idea of the sort of knowledge required in order to interact effectively with patients, but may not be aware that knowledge can in itself set up barriers to properly assessing a patient. Again, this can be dealt with in discussion by asking the group what danger there is in knowing too much about a patient before assessing them. This gives the opportunity to explore the effects of making assumptions before asking an individual to tell his story.

Similarly, when exploring the positive attitudes required, there is often a debate on where the health professional's personal beliefs fit in, particularly if they are dealing with a situation where, for one reason or another, they are not in total accord with the beliefs of their patient.

It can be seen from the above that having an interactive session to identify a common language on effective communication with patients can also bring into the open some of the issues which may not arise in a straight lecture. These include caring for patients with differing belief systems from themselves and the potential problems which may arise. This can form a good basis for the later discussion on support and survival for health professionals, who may want to talk about their needs as individuals as opposed to the needs of those that they care for. In terms of the exercise on common language, it can also help to highlight the non-judgemental element of assessment of patients and families. This brings a sense of reality to a session which may be better remembered than a lecture.

Towards the end of the session the facilitator will need to give a formal summary of the skills, knowledge and attitudes required for effective interaction with patients, relatives and colleagues. This can be achieved in a number of ways:

1. Verbal summary. Here the tutor will refer to the flip chart to give a summary of key points and their importance.
2. Written summary. Here the tutor will list key points on the flip chart in a more relevant order than that gained from the group, thus giving participants a chance to make coherent notes for later study.
3. Hand-out. A hand-out can be very useful in listing key skills with relevant examples. It can be used with a verbal summary and allows participants to concentrate rather than attempt to take notes.

Whichever type of summary is used, time should be allowed for final questions and comments. This gives the facilitator an opportunity to check that the group has made useful connections, but it also allows assurances to be given that further discussion will arise in future sessions when the group will be asked to identify skills in video presentations, audio-tape feedback sessions, and in role play.

SUMMARY

In this chapter there has been emphasis on the importance of a formal session both to set the scene and to recognize the expertise that participants have brought to the course or workshop. Emphasis has been placed on the need to negotiate at all levels on participation and contribution to the work that will be undertaken. It has also been suggested that it may help participants if it is acknowledged that they will occasionally get stuck as they work towards improving their skills.

Guidelines have been given for an interactive session on identifying a common language in terms of the skills, knowledge and attitudes required for effective communication. Such a session will underpin the subsequent content of the course/workshop.

REFERENCE

Faulkner, A. (1992) The evaluation of training programmes for communication skills in palliative care. *Journal of Cancer Care*, **2**, 75–8.

CHAPTER THREE

Using video-taped material

THE VALUE OF VIDEO-TAPED MATERIAL

One of the major values of video-taped material as a teaching tool is that it can be used to demonstrate effective interaction at both verbal and non-verbal levels. It can also be used to demonstrate ineffective interaction and its results. However, it must be remembered that to demonstrate how not to interact with patients should always be followed by another demonstration of how to relate with that patient effectively. If this does not occur, the learning experience can have negative results, perhaps reinforcing inappropriate behaviours.

A demonstration video-tape can also allow for constructive critique in a relatively safe environment. If one compares this with role play, where colleagues are constructively critiquing other colleagues' behaviour, it can be seen that the video-tape is a much safer medium with which to work early in a teaching programme. Through observing effective interaction and constructively suggesting the way forward, the student is not only learning about the skills, knowledge and attitudes required for effective interaction, but is also learning to give feedback in a positive way.

One benefit shared by both video- and audio-taped material is that sections can be replayed if there is any debate or disagreement on what happened in a particular segment. Similarly, the material can be stopped at key points, both to demonstrate good practice, to ask questions of the group about what has happened, to ask the group to predict what might happen as a result of what has gone before, and to allow for interaction between sections of the material.

Video-taped material can be used throughout a teaching programme. Its safety at the beginning of a course has already been noted but another important use is to demonstrate areas of the material that are not generally suitable for other forms of experiential learning. These areas include demonstration of the symptoms of psychiatric morbidity, for example, clinical anxiety and depression, demonstration of interactions with bereaved individuals and demonstration of family issues, particularly if sculpting is not used as a teaching method.

It can be seen that there are many reasons for using video-taped material as part of a teaching programme on effective interaction in health care.

PLANNING A SESSION

A common assumption is that if all else fails, a video is a good 'fall back' for teaching. In fact, video material has to be very carefully considered in terms of group size, the subject to be covered, the material available and the time available. Generally, to be of maximum use, the group should be relatively small, as for other teaching methods in effective interaction. This means that one is looking at a group of 16 to 20 maximum. Video material can, however, be used with a large group but the way in which it is used will differ as will other aspects of the session.

As a general principle, the subject to be covered in a session should dictate whether or not video material is used rather than the reverse. It may be, for example, that at the beginning of a workshop a session is to be held on basic assessment. Given that the language has been agreed and that the group is happy with the skills that they will be observing, the attitudes of the interviewer and the knowledge that they display, then a video on assessment may be considered a suitable medium for the teaching.

It is very important that the tutor is thoroughly familiar with the material to be used, and also gives consideration to the amount of time available for the teaching session. One of the values of video material is that it can be used at a number of levels; for example, it can be used primarily to help students to identify key skills. In this case, the time taken for a session could be relatively short. As a rule of thumb if the video lasts 20 minutes, then it could be shown and key skills discussed in an hour or an hour and a half. If, however, the material is to be used at a more complex level, then more time may be required in order to use the material to demonstrate and to extract from the group the relevant points.

When becoming familiar with the material to be used, it is worth jotting down the specific teaching points that the tutor wishes to make in any session. Some videos come with teaching notes, which suggest stopping points to raise particular points. These are usually guidelines only and certainly do not preclude the tutor from choosing their own teaching points within the material.

Most value seems to be gained from a video if it is stopped at specific points to raise specific issues. For example, if a video were to be shown to demonstrate basic skills, then it may be stopped soon after the opening to demonstrate the way in which the interview has started, whether the interviewer has introduced him/herself, whether they have negotiated over time, taking notes and other important points, and then because that was such a short segment, taking the video back to the start and then running it on again. For later segments, when a stopping point has been debated and the issues identified around it, then the tutor would plan to carry straight on from the stopping point. This pre-planning can ensure that the session (1) has maximum value, and (2) performs the function for which it was planned.

THE SESSION

At the beginning of the session a brief background should be given about the video as should the purpose of the session. Participants should also be invited to take notes. The tutor might introduce the video as follows:

'We are going to show a video this afternoon to demonstrate basic assessment. It's a normal interview that is totally unscripted and so it will have good things in it and it may also have some things in it that you don't like because no-one, even someone described as an expert, gets it right all the time.'

'What we want you to do when watching the video is to note those aspects that you really like in terms of what the interviewer is doing and also to identify the skills that the interviewer is using. I'll be stopping the video from time to time and will be asking you questions about skills used, the non-verbal behaviour and other points that you want to raise. For this reason I suggest that you take some notes of things that are important to you when you are watching this video, and don't forget, when we stop it each time we will be asking you for positive comment first, on what was going well between the interviewer and the patient.'

'This is a lady who has had cancer of the breast and is now dealing with recurrence. The aim of the interviewer is to check out how this lady is coping with the recurrence and what problems she may have as a result.'

After such an introduction, the first segment should be played. Before that, however, it is important to make sure that all participants can see the video-tape clearly. If there are two tutors for the session, then one should concentrate on showing the video and stopping it in the relevant places and the other tutor, although free to make comment throughout the session, takes on the role of screening the group to make sure that nobody is allowed to get distressed without immediate action.

Notes

It is quite useful for the tutor to take notes during each segment so that if there is any query from the participants, then the tutor hopefully will have a note to check out what actually happened. If not, then sections can be replayed, although this will increase the time required for the session. What can be quite surprising is that even with material that the tutors know very well, because they have used it time and time again, there are still new things to be found and identified each time the material is shown. This is particularly important if using the material for more complex discussion because there are shades of meaning to be picked up and different points to be identified.

Stopping points

When the section is stopped the tutor may ask specific questions about skills or non-verbal behaviour, but it is often useful to hand over to the group by asking, 'Any comments?' This more open approach does require that the tutor needs to remind the group that their first comments must be positive, and only after they have been exhausted should constructive suggestions be made about how the interview might have been improved.

If the material is about basic assessment, often the first segment raises all sorts of questions about negotiating time, about taking notes, and about what the patient is called. These can be used as useful teaching points by the tutor who may ask the group how they feel about negotiating time and, indeed, taking notes. This can raise interesting issues where the group may well be split between those who regularly do take notes and those who feel that somehow taking notes can be intrusive. This is one of the big values of a video-tape because the section could then be replayed and the group asked to predict whether indeed the note-taking was getting in the way. If such a question causes puzzlement, then it can be further spelt out by asking how the patient might respond if he or she objected to note-taking.

The issue of negotiating time is again an area of concern to many health professionals. Rather than seeing 20 minutes to half an hour, or whatever has been negotiated, as a reasonable amount of time to give to a patient, they somehow feel that it is insulting by putting some restrictions on time. Again, the group of people themselves would generate considerable discussion on this and the tutor may well have to bring the interaction to a close, perhaps by pointing out what the average time is for any patient with a doctor or a nurse, and then reminding the group that 20 minutes to half an hour is a considerable amount of time. The tutor may then ask the group to predict whether within that time frame the patient will feel free to identify all their current concerns.

If these sort of predictions are made then it is important that, at the end of the video, the tutor goes back and checks out with the group whether their predictions have been fulfilled.

Before moving on to the next segment it is important to screen with the group that they have in fact dealt with all the issues that arose for them from the material. The tutor might say:

'We have established that in that opening segment, which was just a few minutes long, the interviewer has identified her/himself and why she or he is there, s/he has negotiated over time and note-taking, and has asked an open question of the patient to begin to get a picture of this person's perception of their current illness and its background. Some of you, I think, are still not quite convinced that it's all right to negotiate a time and note-taking and we will be coming back to that in other sessions, but I wonder, does anyone want to raise any other issue before we move on to the next segment?'

If there are no further issues to be raised, then the tutor will move on to show the next segment. Each segment will be dealt with in much the same way by identifying the points that the teacher has planned to cover in the session, to pick up specific issues raised by the participants, and to ask the participants to make some predictions about what will happen in the remaining material. Early on in the session it is quite common that several participants have made a contribution and this in itself should encourage quieter members of the group to participate, for they will have seen that comments given are treated with respect and used appropriately.

THE LARGE GROUP

Video-taped material may be shown in a large group but there will be considerable differences in both the way it is shown and the amount of feedback that can be expected from an audience. The size of audience here depends largely on the size of the room and the availability of an enormous screen, and then the participants are very similar to anyone sitting in a cinema; they can see the material, the tutor can stop and start the material and make comments, but it is much less likely that members of the audience will themselves participate.

The situation in the large group is that the tutor is, in effect, giving a lecture with illustrative material. The interaction, if it comes at all from an audience in this situation, is where points in the material cause strong reaction and then someone may make a strong point from the audience. In this case the tutor has to be able to deal with that in a sensitive way. It can be seen that in the large group the tutor has to have a very clear idea of when the video will be stopped, what points will be made and how the session will proceed. Because there will not be so much interaction from the audience, the session will probably be considerably shorter than if that same material was used in a small interactive group.

The problems inherent in showing video material to a large group are those of any straight lecture situation in that there is no way that the tutor can know if the audience is motivated to learn or, indeed, is accepting the points that are being made. There is also an added disadvantage in that if the material is emotional in any way, for example a video-tape on grieving, there is much more chance that people in a large audience will be upset without the opportunity for it to be identified and dealt with. For these reasons, care has to be taken over the choice of material shown to a large audience, and on how the material is handled.

POTENTIAL PROBLEMS

As with any teaching aid, there are inherent problems in using video-taped material. It has been seen that in a large group it may not be possible to screen for adverse reactions to emotionally loaded material. Similarly, in a small group, one has to be concerned about the timing of video-tapes that are likely to evoke strong reactions. If, for example, the material is shown in the last session of the day, then people may go away feeling heavy and upset and not able to discuss those feelings with others. This can have a negative effect on an individual; more seriously, it may have reactivated emotional problems.

If, however, the material is shown earlier in the day, the upset individual will have the chance to talk to someone, perhaps over lunch or a coffee break, and even if their upset is hidden, there is the opportunity for disclosure in other sessions, so that the tutor can make sure that relevant action is taken. Although emotional triggering of this sort is relatively rare, it can be even further reduced if participants are warned that the material is potentially upsetting. Then the tutor can invite anyone who has recently been bereaved, for example, or emotionally upset by someone close to them being ill, to go to the library or to absent themselves from the group. Individuals seldom do this but being given the freedom to do so can alleviate worries in people who are perhaps feeling rather brittle.

Other potential problems may be to do with the material itself and the interviewer and patient on screen. A common question that is raised is whether the patient on screen is real or an actor. The purpose of this question seems to be as much to do with providing an alibi as anything else. It is argued that real patients would not behave like the one on screen, or that real patients would be different in some way. It is important that this question is dealt with in a sensitive but firm way and an exchange about a video-tape where the patient is simulated (see Chapter 5) rather than real, could proceed as follows:

Sally: 'Can I ask if that's a real patient that's being interviewed there?'

Tutor:	'Well, I will tell you Sally, but I wonder why you are asking?'
Sally:	'Well, I thought it may be an actor.'
Tutor:	'What difference do you think it would make if it were an actor?'
Sally:	'Well, I don't think a real patient would be so articulate.'
Tutor:	'Well, is there anybody else concerned here as to whether this is a real patient or an actor?' (A few hands go up and individuals make their own comments about whether this is a real patient.)

'In fact, we do use real patients for these videos but the patient that you are seeing here is what we call a simulated patient. That is, it's somebody who has either been in precisely the situation you've seen or has cared for somebody very close to them who has been in a very similar situation. What these people do for us is to relive their experiences so – no, it's not an actor – yes, it's a patient, but it's a patient who's moved on from the original situation and is reliving it because they want to help others by doing this work. I'll tell you some more about simulators later but I wonder if now we can come back to the video material.'

Another potential problem is that somebody may disagree with what the interviewer is doing. For example, in a video-tape on assessment one of the participants may not particularly like the interviewer's style and then an exchange could go as follows:

Paul:	'I don't like the way the interviewer is pushing this patient along. It's just too fast, she isn't really having a chance to say what she thinks or anything.'
Tutor:	'Can you think of any reason why that could be?'
Paul:	'I think he's just in a hurry and I'm just surprised he's finishing off her words and I'm just not comfortable with it.'
Tutor:	'How do you think the patient feels about this?'
Paul:	'Wouldn't she feel the same too?'
Tutor:	'I'm going to ask this to the whole group. How do you think this lady would behave if she was as irritated as Paul appears to be?'
Joan:	'Well, I think she'd just shut up.'
Tutor:	'You're right. If somebody's interviewing style does not suit a patient, that patient stops disclosing. Now, I can see that you are irritated by this Paul, but in fact I wonder if you can think why this interviewer is moving this lady along?'
Paul:	'I'm not sure.'
Tutor:	'I don't want you to believe me that it's an OK thing to do; what I want you to do is to watch what happens in other

segments of the tape and see if in fact the hurry that you sense now remains, and if so, what is its effect?'

In taking the participant's point and exploring it, the tutor is not laying down rules saying, 'It's OK to move fast', but what the tutor is doing is saying, 'Don't believe that it's OK, but let's see what happens subsequently.'

The tutor is giving the participants a chance to judge the interview by its results, and to explore any areas of concern. It may be, for example, that later in the interview the pace slows as the patient begins to disclose deeper material and concerns, and it is at this point that the tutor could say to Paul, 'Paul, you were pretty irritated at the beginning of this video, I wonder how you're feeling now?'

Paul then has the choice; he can say that he has noticed that the pace has slowed and he is now much happier, or he can maintain his original stance that this is not a style of interviewing that would suit him. In this instance, the tutor would, in a friendly way, agree to differ with the participant. What usually happens, however, is that the participant can see that they were making rather hasty judgements early on and this in itself is a learning experience.

Since Paul is unlikely to have been on his own in these feelings, he does not feel isolated or different – he is a member of a group who is learning and, by definition, not getting it right all the time. The tutor, on the other hand, can reaffirm that the interview is not rehearsed or scripted and that there will be areas where, with hindsight, the interviewer could himself have perhaps been more sensitive, used a slower pace or some other action that would have made the video even better than it is at present.

Another risk with using video material is that the participants will divert attention away from effective interaction on to more physical aspects. For example, there may be some allusion within the material to a particular treatment. Perhaps a patient has been clinically depressed and is not on antidepressants. When the video is next stopped, rather than staying with skills, verbal and non-verbal behaviour, a participant may start asking questions as to why a patient is on tranquillizers when what they would appear to need are antidepressants. It is relatively easy to be drawn into the trap of discussing physical aspects of the material rather than staying with the matter in hand. Alternatively, it is not good to ignore what can be a relevant subject. The interaction here might go as follows:

Adrian: 'I wonder why that lady was not put on antidepressants when we all identified that she had got clinical depression and that view seemed to be shared by the interviewer?'

Tutor: 'You are quite right, Adrian. At the end of the last segment I had asked you to predict whether this lady was depressed

and you all predicted that she was, and indeed we all
agreed that. We are now seeing her in a different setting two
weeks on when her pain is under control and also she tells
us she is on diazepam. Can anyone think of how this change
came about without antidepressants?'

Jim: 'Well, maybe the pain and depression were in fact linked.
We had a patient like that who was depressed but once the
pain was under control, the depression lifted and our lady
didn't even need any tranquillizers.'

Tutor: 'So here we've got yet another mix of treatment. I want to
leave that now because this session is not about treatment
options, but I think that the one thing we can take from it is
that in this second segment of the video this lady has asked
to talk to somebody about her current state and it's quite
obvious from the first segment that we've seen that she's
well able to do that, and that is what is important, rather
than what her doctor gave her for her depression.'

Other problems may involve individual members of the group. It may be
that one or two members have been very quiet throughout the material
and said very little. This is not necessarily a problem. Some participants
are quiet and may not say anything on the first day. It is only if they re-
main quiet on subsequent days that the tutor would expect to have a
quiet word with them to see if there are any difficulties. There are also
individuals who may be just a little over-eager and in that instance it is
sometimes worth saying, 'That's a really good point you've made and
you are obviously very interested in this material, but I wonder if other
people would like to add anything to this?' This is a sensitive way of
letting someone know that they are taking rather too much of the floor.

Just occasionally someone may be quite disruptive within the group
and a decision has to be made then as to whether this disruption is due
to upset or whether it is a deliberate ploy to gain attention. These and
other problems will be discussed in Chapter 8.

THE VALUE OF PRODUCING MATERIAL

There are a number of videos available on communication and
counselling. These are listed on page 135. However, many tutors feel that
they would like to make their own material for demonstration. The value
of this is that it allows the tutor to demonstrate their own skills while still
being able to give attention to the group, and it means that early on in
the course or workshop, participants are encouraged to critique
interactions at 'one removed'. In addition, the tutor will be able to
answer any questions about, for example, why a particular drug regimen

was used or, more pertinently in communication terms, why they took a particular line of enquiry, or why they missed one cue and followed another. Such a situation allows for a session that is totally reality based.

In showing material that includes oneself, the tutor is demonstrating that it is all right to not get things right, and this is really important because if the tutor is seen to be too perfect, then this can have a deskilling effect on the participants in the group. If, on the other hand, the tutor can say, 'Yes, with hindsight I would not have done that. Can anyone suggest what I could have done?', then they are demonstrating their own vulnerability.

To make video-taped material, however, access is required to a studio where the material can be made, and to patients, simulators or actors. Some of these might carry a cost. For example, a university audio-visual department may well seek a charge for making material unless the tutor is on the staff of that university. The alternative is to use a video camera and to literally make one's own material. The problem with this is that the quality is likely to be poor and this can be off-putting to participants who are used to broadcast-quality material.

For those tutors wishing to make their own material, the first step would be to make enquiries about studios in the area, either in colleges of technology or universities, and then to approach those people and ask for help. If funding is required, drug firms may be interested. What has to be observed here is whether there would be any strings to that funding. The firm, for example, may want to promote a drug on the video, which means that the tutor who is making the material will, by definition, become associated with that drug and be seen to approve its use.

For the tutor who feels that material is required that is not readily available, but who does not want to go into the mechanics of making their own, then the opportunity they have is to alert a company that is known to make videos on the new material that is required. Help the Hospices, for example, has funded videos that are widely used both in this country and abroad. The drug firm Pfizer has also made videos for distribution throughout the country.

SUMMARY

It has been seen in this chapter that video-taped material is a valuable resource in both demonstrating effective and ineffective interaction and for demonstrating areas that are more difficult to cover using other experiential methods. It has value because it can be replayed, it can be stopped at key points and it can be used by both small and large groups.

Sessions using video-tapes should be carefully planned, taking into consideration the group number, the subject to be covered, the material available and the time available. Tutors should familiarize themselves with the material and plan in advance what particular teaching points they are going to make.

Students should understand the purpose of the session and be invited to take notes so that they can properly participate in the session. The video should be played in segments, with questions and comments between each section. Although superb for interactive sessions, the video material may also be used for a large group to illustrate a lecture on a particular area.

Potential problems should be foreseen, which include the nature of the material in that if it is emotional it may trigger reactions in participants, that participants may use the material to disagree with the tutor or to move away from communication to technical and physical matters, and to alibi if they feel that the patient is somehow not real. Individual reactions should be observed to pick up any distress within the group.

Although there are a number of video-tapes available (see page 135), there is some value in tutors making their own material and this should be made as a result of enquiries in the tutor's own locality as to what is on offer. Simple material may be made with a video machine, but the quality is likely to be very inferior to that of company-produced material.

CHAPTER FOUR

Role play

Role play as a teaching method can be very potent since it allows practice in a relatively safe environment. Unfortunately, members of the group may have had experience of badly managed role play and others may be very apprehensive about being involved. For this reason, prior to setting up role play sessions, it is essential to give clear guidelines to the group on safety strategies which will operate, and to contract with the group on their involvement. Before deciding to use role play as a teaching method, several considerations need to be addressed, including the time available, size of the group and the suitability of the material to be covered.

SAFETY STRATEGIES

Positive feedback

It is useful to start the session by asking for participants to share previous experiences of role play, and to discuss reasons why some participants have enjoyed it while others have not. Then some reassurance can be given that a positive approach will be taken, that is, that first feedback on what has happened in role play will put emphasis on what has gone well. Only when the positives have been exhausted will constructive suggestions be allowed for improved performance. The penalty for negative criticism is that the critical student must suggest an improved strategy from the one that they have criticized.

Time out

Time out is a mechanism that allows a role player to stop the role play without any feelings of guilt. The rationale for this is to remind the students that they would only be doing the role play if the situation was one in which they found difficulty. This means that at some point in the role play it is very likely that the player who is interviewing will get stuck.

As a teacher it is important to let the students know that this is appreciated and that no student will be allowed to wallow, unknowing what to do in a particular situation. Students should be encouraged to use their own mechanism for asking for time out. They may say, 'I'm stuck', or, 'Help', or, 'What on earth do I do now?'

Sometimes, even when the tutor has made it explicit that time out is a reasonable thing to ask for, the student will stay in a situation which is becoming difficult to handle. When negotiating the ground rules for role play, the tutor should point out that she will on occasion stop the role play, either to give a student time out or because of a particular teaching point that needs to be made. As a tutor it is important to emphasize that when a student is stuck, that student alone will not be asked to generate ways of moving forward, but that the responsibility for this will rest with the group.

The role

When an area to be explored through role play has been agreed by the group, then volunteers should be recruited who have had a similar situation to deal with. For example, if the area is that of breaking bad news, then the group will be asked if anyone in that group has found difficulty with breaking bad news.

When participants have been identified, one of them will be asked to volunteer to play the person who received the bad news and someone else will be asked if they would interview that person. It will be explained to the group that to make the task manageable each player will stay in their own basic skin, that is they will not change sex, age or their social circle, but will put the elements of the role to be played into their normal persona.

This 'own skin' approach does cut down on the likelihood of comments that role play is not real and is rather silly. Both players are then free to concentrate on the elements of their role without having to think of age or infirmity.

No personal experience

There are many reasons why people will agree to participate in role play, and not just that they wish to practise in a relatively safe environment. One very potent reason for wishing to take on a role is to deal with personal problems that are very closely related to the task.

For this reason it should be made quite explicit when setting out the rules of role play that no-one should volunteer to take on a role that is 'too close to home'. To do so would run the risk of triggering (which will be discussed in detail in Chapter 8), which can be counterproductive rather than the catharsis that the player may have hoped for.

Making the task explicit

The group should be reassured at each role play that the task to be undertaken will be made quite explicit in the briefing, and that no-one will be put in a situation where they are unaware of the task they have in hand. Although this may sound controlling, it is a very important part of maintaining safety within the group. It gives each role player the sure knowledge that they are not going to have to manufacture a task in a difficult situation under the scrutiny of the rest of the group, and it also gives the group the feeling of safety that they know exactly what they are undertaking in any particular role play interaction.

Responsibility

Another safety factor for the players which should be explained is that when the role play is stopped, either by one of the players or by the tutor, that the responsibility for discussion and suggestions for moving forward will be asked for from the group. This makes it explicit that the role play is a whole-group experience and that people who take on specific roles within the session will not also be expected to get themselves out of the 'hot water' that they were worried about. It also puts the teacher into the role of facilitator and, to a certain extent, it mimics the real life situation of talking to patients who are encouraged to generate their own solutions to problems rather than to have edicts from health care workers. Figure 4.1 summarizes these ground rules.

NEGOTIATING WITH THE GROUP

When the safety rules have been made explicit, then it is possible to move on and negotiate with the group that they will in fact take part in the role play.

Size of group

In negotiating it is important to look at the size of the group. Role play in a large group can have difficulties, both in terms of what is expected from the players, how much feedback it is possible to get from the group and the enhanced risk of triggering (page 79) that can occur. The ideal group for role play is eight to ten participants, but it is possible with one tutor to go up to 12 people.

With eight to ten participants the responsibility for the role play and its progression rests on six to eight people, which means that no-one feels under any particular pressure. Too small a group can cause pressure on both the players and the two or three people who are observing them, while too large a group can cause problems in terms of

1. Emphasis will be on positive feedback, i.e. what is going well

2. Constructive suggestions for improvement will be made rather than negative criticism

3. 'Players' are free to call 'time out' at any time, rather than struggle on with a difficult situation where they may 'get stuck'

4. The tutor will call 'time out' if the scenario gets too difficult, or to reinforce good practice

5. At 'time out' points the *group* will be asked to generate possible strategies for the player to select and try, rather than the player who is 'stuck'

6. The 'patient' will be asked to follow a clear brief and not make it harder for the interviewer than has been agreed

7. No-one will play a part that is 'too close to home'

8. All players will stay in their own skins (no sex or age change)

9. All members of the group will be expected to take part

10. All scenarios will be based on participant's current clinical practice

Figure 4.1 Safety rules for role play.

participation and the temptation for free-loading within the session. Further, the tutor has difficulty in screening the whole group.

Time

Role play is not an activity that can be just slotted in to a programme as a 'one off'. It often is used in that way but can be quite damaging because the tutor may not see the group again and may not know if somebody has been hurt by the experience. Time for role play should include time to pick up any pieces where people have been upset to any degree by the activity.

A rule of thumb is that if a tutor has a group for half a day or less, role play is really not appropriate or safe to use. If the tutor has a longer time, then what needs to be negotiated is how much time there is for the activity so that everyone can take part.

Contracting

It is useful to make a verbal contract with the group that they will all take part in role play. Having negotiated the amount of time available for role play, it should be possible to agree that everyone will take part even if it is not until the next session a week later. By negotiating in this way, everyone feels equally involved.

Occasionally there may be a group that is not going to get together long enough for everybody to have a chance to role play. In this situation, unless a firm contract is made, it could be that the participants wait for everyone else to volunteer knowing that all the group will not be able to participate.

A very effective way to deal with this, which brings an element of humour into decision making, is to put it to the group that, unfortunately, there is not enough time for everyone to be involved. The tutor needs to work out how many people can be involved, take a piece of paper for each member of the group and mark with a cross enough pieces to gain enough role players for the time in hand.

A contract is then made with the group that those who take a piece of paper with a cross on are the lucky ones who will be allowed to role play, and those who have a blank sheet will agree not to be too cross that they do not have a chance. This usually gains a considerable amount of laughter and goodwill towards the exercise and relaxes any tension.

Focus of role play

The best role plays are usually those that have a direct relationship to problems that participants have found in their own clinical reality. If an agenda has been agreed then common problems will have been identified. The tutor needs to look at the priority list and decide which scenarios are suitable for practise in role play. If an agenda has not been set, participants can be asked to offer scenarios at the start of the session.

Some problems lend themselves very well to role play. These include dealing with anger, answering difficult questions, breaking bad news, basic assessment and other areas where the practitioner has a chance to actually practise skills.

Some areas may be seen to be unsuitable for role play; family situations for example, where four or five people need to be briefed, are quite difficult to handle if there is only one tutor, and the time taken to brief each member of the family would mean that the session would be over long. It would also be quite difficult for the observers to take in all the dynamics of the interaction. Another area that is quite difficult and has to be handled with extreme care is that of bereavement. This is one of the areas where it is very easy to trigger unhappy experiences in the group and also to have the whole group feeling quite low after what is a very draining experience.

The final decision on whether the material is suitable for role play has to rest with each individual tutor, and much will depend on previous experience of running such a group and managing the dynamics of that group.

Gaining volunteers

Before actually asking for volunteers, two points can be made that will have some influence on people's decision to volunteer sooner rather than later.

(a)   Hierarchy of difficulty

It can be pointed out to the group that the initial role plays will be in relatively simple areas such as basic assessment. This can motivate some members of the group to volunteer sooner rather than later in the hope that they will have a more manageable task than the difficult ones which will come later. This strategy does have an element of humour because almost always one member of the group will interpret the message as gentle blackmail.

(b)   Value of experience

Here the tutor points out the value of having a chance to experience a situation that has been found to be difficult, so that group members can begin to relate to some of the feelings of the patient or relative. Second, the tutor points out the value to the person who is in their own professional role, since they too are having the chance to practise in a relatively safe environment where they know that they can bale out if things get too difficult. The support, help and suggestions from the rest of the group can also reassure the player so that he or she can practise a number of strategies in a relatively safe environment.

Before asking for volunteers, the tutor should remind the group of the focus of the particular role play. It might be, for example, that the focus is breaking bad news and the tutor might say to the group, 'Is there anyone here who has had to break bad news recently and feels that somehow it could have gone better?' This will usually elicit responses from more than one member of the group. The tutor would then say, 'Well, there are two or three of you that had this experience; which one of you would like to be the person who is going to receive the bad news?' The skill then is in waiting for a volunteer and making maximum use of silence. Inevitably someone will break it by saying, for example, 'Oh well, I suppose I might as well get it over.'

The tutor should then address the rest of the group and say, 'Is there anyone who would like to be the interviewer, the person who is going to break bad news?' As with the first volunteer, silence will usually elicit someone who says, 'I had trouble breaking bad news to someone. Could I have a go?' In the unlikely event of no-one offering to play the role, one strategy that does work is to ask the group which of them had given priority to breaking bad news as an issue they wished to cover. This will often be followed by one of those people saying, 'OK, I'll do it.'

The tutor needs to remember that in a group which has not been involved in role play before with this particular tutor, a good deal of trust is required all round, and the volunteers should be thanked for being the first to take on roles.

BRIEFING

The success of role play depends largely at this point on really clear briefing of both the players and of the group, and in setting up the group so that the players are distanced from the group by the space of perhaps two or three chairs (Figure 4.2).

The health professional should be put into the chair where they will interview, and asked to get into their professional skin, and begin to

Role players

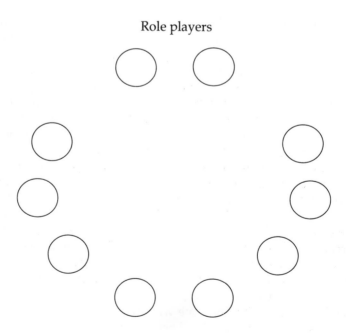

Figure 4.2 Grouping of chairs for role play.

think of how they will handle the task. The participant taking the role of the patient or relative is taken outside for briefing.

Briefing the 'patient'

There are a number of points to consider when briefing someone for the role of patient.

(a)   *Reality base*

The player should be asked to remember a real experience in their own clinical practice where breaking bad news was a difficulty for them. They should be asked to give a 'thumb nail' sketch of the problem as they perceived it and encouraged to give the major points of the case study they are presenting. The tutor can then take the strands from this and give a brief to the player of the sort of patient they are to play and the situation that they are to portray. The exchange may go as follows:

Tutor: 'You will remember that this is a bad news situation; can you give me a brief outline of a bad news situation that you found a little difficult?'

Player: 'Yes I can. It was a patient in the hospice. He'd come in for respite care; his wife had been looking after him pretty well day and night and was exhausted. It was one of those sad things that within 12 hours of being admitted, he just died and I had to tell his wife.'

Tutor: 'OK, so you're going to be that wife. You need to think yourself into how it was when you were looking after your husband; how tired you got, all the things you've been telling me and to be unsure why the hospice has telephoned you and asked you to come and see sister. Do you think you can get into those sorts of feelings?'

Player: 'Oh yes, yes. When I talk about her I can remember that woman and how apprehensive she was when she came in to my office.'

Tutor: 'Before we develop this any further, can I ask you whether this situation is going to be too near to home for your comfort.'

Player: 'Oh no, no. I'm lucky. Nobody that I care about has died in the whole of my lifetime.'

Tutor: 'Well, if you get yourself into the feelings that you observed in this wife who was going to get bad news, incorporate it into your own skin, your own social life, so that you don't have to remember all the relatives etc. of that person. I want you to react to what comes to you, so be led by the interviewer, and if you feel that the person is breaking the bad news in a way that you can accept, then don't feel that you mustn't accept it. The big thing is that you take the bad news in the way that it comes across to you and that you do not make the situation any more difficult than it has to be.'

Player: 'I think I understand that.'

Tutor: 'Any more questions?'

Player: 'No, no. I'm going to be the wife. My husband's been in the hospice just 12 hours; I've had a telephone call to come to the hospice, and I'm just not sure what it's all about and I'm a bit frightened inside, and I'm feeling exhausted because I haven't had much sleep in the last week or two.'

Tutor: 'That sounds fine – and, remember, don't make it any more difficult than it has to be.'

Briefing the professional

The player who is going to be the patient in this role play is taken back into the room, sat in one of the role playing chairs and asked to get into role, to think themselves into the role that they are portraying. The professional is then taken out of the room to be briefed.

It is important to give the professional an outline of the situation to be portrayed and to ask the player if dealing with that situation is going to cause any problems for them. Occasionally a professional might say, 'Well, actually it's a bit close to home for me. I haven't actually had bad news that somebody I loved had died, but I did recently have some bad news of a different sort, and now that I think of it I'm a little bit uncomfortable.'

In this instance, it is important to take the professional back into the group and to say quite clearly, 'In discussing this role we find that Julie isn't the best person to play it. Can we have another volunteer?' No-one should be pressured into fulfilling a role that is likely to trigger unpleasant reactions within them.

When the professional has agreed the task and has been screened to make sure that they are not going to be damaged by it, then the task has to be made absolutely explicit once again. The tutor might say something like, 'Julie, I want you to remember that your primary aim here is to break bad news. That's quite difficult but don't be led aside from that main task. You remember that the wife has had her husband admitted just over 12 hours ago to give her a break. She's been very, very tired because she's been looking after him day and night with little help, and you have to break to her the news that her husband has died quite unexpectedly.

'You will remember that the basic principle is that you fire a warning shot and then break the bad news, and we'll see how it goes from there. Have you any questions?'

Player: 'No, no. I think I'm all right.'

The tutor should then remind the player of the safety rules; that they are able to call time out, and that they will not be expected to generate solutions to their own problems, but that if they want to contribute ideas, then there will be no reason why they should not do that. The important thing is in letting the player know that they are not being put into a 'hot seat' situation.

Before taking the professional back into the rest of the group it is worth discussing with them what their opening gambit might be. The tutor can offer an opening gambit, but it is better if the player is allowed to choose their own, and the tutor will offer one only if asked. For example:

Tutor: 'Julie, do you want to think of how you're going to open the interaction? You'll remember that Mrs Brown has come at your request to your office to find out how things are with her husband.'

Julie: 'Well, I thought I'd bring her into my office, ask her to sit down and then tell her that I've got some serious news for her.'

Tutor: 'That sounds like a good warning shot. Are you happy to go in now?'

Julie: 'Oh yes. Let's get it over with (laughing).'

THE ROLE PLAY

Before starting the role play, it is worth reminding the group of the positive feedback mechanism and other safety rules, to remind the players in front of the group that they are able to take time out when they want to but that there may be points when the tutor will stop the role play.

It is then important to give the group a brief resumé of the situation. The tutor might say, 'Jill is playing the role of Mrs Brown, who's been looking after her dying husband on her own at home for a considerable number of weeks. The district nurse, calling in to see how things were, found that Mrs Brown was exhausted and she persuaded Mrs Brown to let her husband go into the local hospice for respite care. Unfortunately, Mr Brown died after he had been in the hospice for 12 hours. The sister has phoned Mrs Brown asking her if she will come in to the hospice to see her. Julie is the sister and she has the task of breaking bad news to Mrs Brown.'

Once the scene has been set in this way, the group needs to be given clear directives as to their part in the role play. The tutor may say, for example, 'The role play will not be allowed to run for too long because, even in a short piece of role play, there will be lots of points for discussion and for learning. Your role is to observe the interaction, looking for what you find most effective, and making some points as to how you think the interaction might be improved. You will probably need to take some notes so that you remember the points that you want to discuss. I'm going to ask Julie to start as soon as she feels ready, and then either we will stop when Julie wants some time out or I may stop it if there's a particular teaching point that seems important.'

After this introduction, which has given the role players time to get into role and think about what they are going to do, the tutor should take a seat either separate from the group but where she can scan both the role players and the group, or some teachers prefer to stand behind the group, again so that they can see the interactions that are going on and also the reactions of the group to the role play.

Stop points

(a)   Time out

The most usual reason for a player calling time out is because he/she feels that they just do not know what to do next. They may say, 'I'm getting stuck' or 'I don't know what to do' or 'I'm just feeling over-whelmed by this.' The tutor should legitimize this need for time out and then, giving the player a chance to get over the feeling that things are going badly, the tutor should ask the group to give some very positive feedback to the interviewer on what has gone well so far. The group may pick up a good introduction, open questions or the skills being used, and this will help to give the interviewer a feeling that positive progress is being made. Only when all the positives have been exhausted should the tutor ask the group to make constructive suggestions (rather than criticisms) for the way forward.

The aim of this approach is to generate a number of strategies that may or may not work, that involve the whole group. The tutor's role is to put a value on everything that is offered. Sometimes this is not easy because the solution offered patently would not work. Rather than saying that to a group member, it is better to ask the group, 'Well that's one possibility, but I wonder if anybody could think why it might not work?' In this way, discussion is generated about the ideas put forward rather than individual members of the group feeling that they have said something silly.

When a number of strategies has been suggested, the interviewer is asked to choose one of those strategies that they would like to try and see if it works for them. The role play then continues with the tutor suggesting a start point to get back into the interaction. Only if there are no ideas at all from the group should the tutor offer strategies at this point.

(b)   Teaching points

Sometimes an interviewer will be getting into the role play and will be doing things that are absolutely effective for the particular situation. The way it is progressing may be so good that the teacher wants to stop the role play and ask the group why she has actually stopped it. Given that group members can pick up what was going so well, there is reinforcement both for the interviewer at an almost immediate level, but also reinforcement for the group in that they are able to pick up and identify the effective strategies that are being demonstrated.

Some people believe that teaching points can also be negative, that is, the tutor can stop the role play to talk about what has gone wrong. If this strategy is used it must be used in a very sensitive manner and, rather than asking what is going wrong in the role play, it would be better if the tutor asked for positive feedback as usual, and then followed it with, 'I wonder if anyone can think of something that may be more effective than the point at which I stopped the role play?' This leaves the interviewer feeling that they were not doing anything particularly wrong, simply that there is a better way to do it that, with hindsight, the group may identify.

Taking this approach reminds both the players and the group that the aim of role play is to build on existing strengths rather than to destroy people's self-confidence. This also has the effect of helping potential role players to feel safe enough to volunteer for future sessions.

(c)   Player in difficulties

Just as the teacher may stop role play to make a teaching point, there is also a responsibility to stop the role play if it is obvious that the interviewer is beginning to get into difficulties. By stopping in this way and asking the group first for positive feedback and then for constructive suggestions, the interviewer is saved from getting into a terribly difficult situation that they feel embarrassed about.

Again, the tutor does not need to make explicit that the stopping point is because of potential difficulties, but she may ask the interviewer how they felt the interview was going. Often the response is one of relief that time out has been called and the interviewer may say, 'I felt that I was somehow getting into a problem, but I just hoped it would sort itself out.'

From this it can be seen that all role players are not able to ask for time out as soon as they feel difficulties arise, and that is why the tutor has to take this particular responsibility and use it in a positive and reinforcing way.

Focus

If the role players have a clear brief, then hopefully the role play will stay in focus. However, it is possible for the group members to pick up on points that are not to do with the focus of the role play. There are a number of reasons why the focus may not be maintained.

(a)   Role player effect

The role player may go off the point of their brief. For example, Mary was given the role of the wife who was going to receive bad news. She would then be surprised and distressed when sister told her that her husband was dead. Mary might in fact react with extreme anger, and if the tutor does not bring the role play back in focus, then the discussion at stopping points may be a lot more about dealing with anger than it is to do with breaking bad news.

The role player may also be making this situation too difficult. This does occur when the person who has offered to play the role was not able themselves to deal with the situation, and it may be that at an unconscious level they do not want a colleague in role play to do better than they did in real life.

The tutor can deal with the above points by making explicit what is happening, not in any critical way but by simply pointing out that although anger may be a reaction to bad news, this is something that will be addressed in a later role play. Then it is possible to return to the focus of how to break bad news.

In the situation where the role is made too difficult, the tutor needs to acknowledge the problems for someone who has had to accept that they do not always get things right, and that there is a temptation in all of us to try and make sure that nobody else gets it right either. This can cause some light-hearted remarks as long as it is put across in a positive acknowledging way.

(b)   Alibis

It can happen in a role play that the person who is interviewing gets into difficulties. When the tutor asks the group to look at what has been happening, the group will begin to present alibis as to why the interviewer could not do anything different. The tutor's role here is to pick up each alibi and to ask the group what is happening so that they themselves take responsibility for coming back to the real issue of effective strategies, and come to the realization that in making alibis for non-effective communication, they are defeating the purpose of the role play.

(c)   Differing views

When a tutor stops role play for whatever reason and asks for positive comments, very often the response is more to do with assumptions about what is happening in the interaction than in terms of the skills and strategies being used. For example, in the bad news situation, rather than giving positive feedback on opening gambits or questioning style or other aspects of the interaction, members of the group may begin to make assumptions about what is happening. They may, for example, say that it is not possible for sister to make the leap from introduction to bad news because of how obviously apprehensive the relative is.

The above comment is partly alibi but very much to do with making assumptions. If this is then thrown open to the whole group, other members may interpret the role-playing relative as having very different emotions. When this happens, the tutor should use the situation to remind the group that one should not make any assumption without some information to back it up.

EFFECT OF ROLE PLAY ON THE GROUP

In taking a role play session, it is important to monitor the players and the group as well as possible. It is also important to ask the group from time to time through the role play how they are feeling.

In the 'breaking bad news' role play, the group may feel quite affected by the distress of the person playing the bereaved relative, so the tutor should ask not only the patient how they are feeling, to monitor for triggering and for distress, but also the group.

If the group admits, or individuals within the group admit, that they are feeling upset by what they are seeing, then the tutor should legitimize those feelings. Too often, health professionals feel that they have to be tough and not show feelings; in fact, the tutor can point out that if health professionals do not react at some level, then it means that they are not connecting with the people they care for.

Sometimes a group feels quite cross with the tutor for stopping role play at particular points. They may argue that the flow is lost and that it is not fair to the role players. The tutor should point out the reasons for short segments of role play, and the benefits to be gained from them, and also clarify with the role players that they are able to come in and out of role without to much difficulty. Most people in role welcome stopping points to reassure them, and also to give them a chance to consider new and more effective strategies.

CONCLUDING

There has to be enough time left at the end of role play to summarize what has happened, to underline the teaching points, and to thank the role players for their effort and the group for their good involvement in the session.

Importantly, the players should be debriefed. This does not normally require them walking up and down saying who they are and what they are not, but simply asking them if they are comfortably out of role and observing them. If there is any sign of upset, then this should be taken up privately with them.

If the role play has gone well, then the group should be feeling very happy to go on with more role play or discussion, and will themselves say how useful they have found the session. By having asked the group how they were feeling, it should be possible to identify any problems that may have arisen.

SUMMARY

In this chapter, role play has been considered as a potent teaching strategy which requires careful negotiation with participants in order that it becomes as safe an activity as possible.

Preparation includes the setting and agreeing of ground rules in negotiation with the group, and a contractual arrangement for all, or as many as possible, to take part.

The most successful scenarios are those based on clinical problems offered by group members, with emphasis on positive feedback and constructive suggestion.

CHAPTER FIVE

The use of audio feedback

Many research studies, for example, Faulkner (1992), Faulkner and Maguire (1983), Maguire, Faulkner and Fairburn (1989), have all shown that audio feedback on communication skills can be a very potent learning exercise. These studies have used audio feedback as a means of measuring skills from a transcript after an interaction has taken place. However, in this chapter audio feedback will be considered as a means of teaching students how to improve their communication skills.

PLANNING

As with other experiential teaching methods, the group size is one of the first considerations, since every student needs to have some feedback of their own material. This allows for interest and for a positive approach to be maintained since everyone knows that they will be involved. In general terms, the group size should be similar to that for other skills-based learning, such as role play. This means a group of no more than eight to ten people for one tutor, but if the group is larger, then providing there are tutors for each eight to ten participants, that group can be split into small groups for feedback.

Another consideration when planning to use audio feedback as a teaching method is the number of sessions that will be given to this exercise and the length of each session that can be given. In a session of one and a half hours, to give due attention to participants, it is unlikely that more than three audiotapes could be discussed. This means that for a group of ten, then at least five hours would have to be available for this exercise.

One could argue that every participant will learn from the exercise whether or not their own material is heard, but it is much more potent if each student can have feedback on at least part of their audio-taped interaction. A rule of thumb is that audio feedback should be used only if every member of the group can have adequate feedback and a chance to give feedback to their colleagues. However, this is not written on tablets of stone and it may be that the tutor has to decide that, due to time constraints, every participant will have a chance for some feedback but some may gain it through participating in role play while others gain it through bringing recordings of interactions with their patients. Alternatively, the tutor may decide in planning a course to use only one of these two options.

Perhaps one of the most important considerations when planning an audio feedback session is to decide how the tape-recorded interviews are to be made. There are two main options: (1) to ask each participant to record an interaction with a patient or relative of their choice and (2) to arrange for simulated interviews to be made as part of the work of the course.

Interviews in the clinical session

At first sight, it might seem that making a tape recording of an interview with a patient, if that patient gave informed consent, is the best possible option. It eliminates the chance to alibi that the situation is not real and, therefore, the participant cannot behave in the way they normally would. It also allows the participant to record an interview with a patient with whom they feel comfortable and at a time when it is convenient for them.

In day-release courses at Trent Palliative Care Centre, it has been found that there are difficulties in asking participants, be they doctors, nurses or social workers, to record interactions with their own patients. The main problems identified have been as follows:

1. There were no suitable patients around at a time when the tape recording could have been made;
2. The patient, or sometimes relative, that has been chosen has been totally unsuitable for the task that has been given;
3. The quality of the tape recordings, given the background noise, has often been so poor that it is impossible to hear the interaction.

Interviews with simulated patients

The use of simulators has been described by Faulkner (1992). Briefly, a simulator is someone who has either had a particular disease or who has nursed somebody, or cared for them, at very close range while they were ill. These people are trained to relive their story in a way that allows a health professional to interview them and gain some perspective of their reactions to diagnosis and prognosis. If simulators are used for audio feedback purposes, then the first part of the course will have to allow for these interviews to take place. The advantages of simulated interviews are as follows:

1. There can be standardization of the level of difficulty experienced by the participant in assessing a patient;

2. The length of the interview can be controlled;
3. The tutor will know the major problems of the patient and have a clear idea of their background. This enables feedback to be much more realistic;
4. The quality of recording can be monitored;
5. There are no difficulties of access to an appropriate patient at an appropriate time.

Once a decision has been made as to whether to use actual or simulated patients for the interviews, then some thought will need to be given before the session on how the participants are going to be briefed and how they are going to be sure to be co-operative. If, for example, briefing is to be written so that students can make their tape recordings before they come, then clear notes will need to be made so that each participant knows precisely what is expected of them (Figure 5.1). If the interaction

---

Before you interview your patient, please read the following briefing notes, and practise using the tape recorder with a friend.

1. Your task is to interview a patient with the aim of assessing current problems

2. Please choose a patient who has been recently admitted to your ward, or referred for a home visit

3. You need to gain informed consent from the patient and should explain that you wish to record your interview so that you can get feedback on your skills, and so improve the way you work with patients

4. If the patient consents, offer confidentiality, and explain that the recording will be used only for teaching purposes

5. Your interview should last for no more than 20 minutes, and should be recorded in its entirety

6. Please listen to your interview after it is complete and choose two parts of it to share with the group:

   (a) The part where you felt most confident;

   (b) The part (if any) where you felt that you could be more effective.

7. If you have any difficulty, please telephone me at the centre.

Figure 5.1 Briefing notes for audio-taped assessments.

is to be made with a simulated patient, then the tutor will need to have clear notes so that the group can be briefed as to what is expected of them.

In terms of ensuring that participants are co-operative and will submit to having an audio-tape of their interaction made, whether with a real or simulated patient, it is important to plan some form of contracting with the whole group prior to the session when the audio feedback is introduced as one of the potential teaching methods.

Finally, some thought must be given to resources in that if there are a group of 20 students with two tutors, that means in effect 20 tape recorders. Few institutes of education have that number of resources, but it is usually safe to assume that many of the participants will have good tape recorders of their own. This leads to a decision on the minimum number of tape recorders required to cover the needs of the group. It is usually possible to have one tape recorder between two, three or even four students if they are going to interview actual patients and have a reasonable length of time to do it. They can then take responsibility for handing the tape recorder on and for organizing the interviews so that they do not all need the machine on the same day.

If, on the other hand, simulated patients are to be interviewed, then the considerations in terms of resources will have to be the number of rooms required and a similar number of tape recorders. Figure 5.2 shows a typical layout of simulated interviews with a group over a period of time. The more rooms and tape recorders that are available, the faster the interviews will be able to be made but, in addition to the rooms and the tape recorders, there also needs to be helpers who will see participants in and out of the room in which they are to do their interview, who will switch on recorders, give instructions and monitor the exercise.

INTRODUCING AUDIO FEEDBACK TO PARTICIPANTS

The tutor will need to introduce the subject of audio feedback as a means of learning in a very positive and constructive way. As with the introduction of role play to a group, this must be done with absolute confidence that the group will co-operate. Having chosen the method of recording, that is, actual or simulated patients, this should be negotiated with the group, with time given for participants to raise questions and concerns. Probably few participants, if any, will have been asked to tape record interactions before so there may be quite a lot of concern about the use of tape recorders. Even in 1993 many individuals have not heard their own voice on audio or video tape and this may be another concern. Each concern raised by a participant should be considered seriously and discussed with the group, while holding to the notion that the learning

Time	Rooms			
	134	111	Boardroom	Quiet room
9.45 Patient	A. Brown (D1) Mr Radford	T. Fox (D2) Ms Jones	M. Murray (D3) Ms Parker	B. Bird (D4) Mr Hutchin
10.15 Patient	O. Bright (D5) Mrs Kirk	S. Rowe (D6) Mr Williams	P. Sands (D7) Mr Pearce	H. Owens (D8) Ms West
10.45 Patient	P. Byron (D9) Mr Radford	C. Airds (D10) Ms Jones	A. Black (D11) Ms Parker	T. Jones (D12) Mr Hutchin
11.15 Patient	R. Windsor (D13) Mrs Kirk	J. Peacock (D14) Mr Williams	F. Cater (D15) Mr Pearce	W. Woods (D16) Ms West

Group A	Group B
(Agenda set 9.45–10.45) (Interviews 10.45–11.45)	(Interviews 9.45–10.45) (Agenda set 10.45–11.45)
P. Bryon C. Airds A. Black T. Jones R. Windsor J. Peacock F. Cater W. Woods	A. Brown T. Fox M. Murray B. Bird O. Bright S. Rowe P. Sands H. Owens

Figure 5.2 Typical schedule for audio-taped assessments.

potential is such that the tutor is confident of full co-operation from the group.

It could be maintained that many participants would be very much against the idea of having an interview with a patient audio-taped, but in a study aimed to evaluate workshops on communication and counselling in cancer and palliative care (Faulkner, 1992) there were only two refusals among more than 200 participants. These participants comprised doctors, nurses, social workers and one or two members of the clergy.

Once the notion of audio feedback has been accepted by a group, the tutor needs to contract with the group that everybody will take part. This will be more readily accepted if the contract includes confidentiality, clear agreement on the use of the audio-tapes and reinforcement of the fact that feedback will focus on what is going well in the interview and that only when all the good points have been discussed will constructive suggestion be made by the group.

USE OF THE AUDIO-TAPES

In Maguire and Faulkner's study (Faulkner, 1992), it was necessary to contract with the group that the audio-tapes would be used to measure their skills at the beginning, the end and at follow-up of their workshop. Promises were given that the audio-tapes would not be heard by anyone except members of the research team. When using audio-taped interviews for feedback, similar promises should be given that the only people who will hear the audio-tapes are the group and the tutors, and that after use they will either be given back to the participant or they will be blanked out for use on further courses. Audio-taped interviews should only have wider use, that is, for teaching purposes elsewhere, with the full permission of the interviewer and interviewee.

Part of the contract will also include the use of the audio-tape in the teaching session. If there is half an hour for each participant and they have each made a 20-minute tape, then it becomes apparent that only part of their tape can be heard. Wherever possible, the decision on which part of the tape to share with the group and the tutor should be made by the participant. If, for example, all the interviews are made on one morning and the following week feedback begins to three of the participants, then there is time for them to take home their tape-recording to listen to and pick out, first, that part of the audio-tape with which they were most pleased and, second, the part of the tape with which they were much less pleased.

Group members will also be expected to contract that feedback to their colleagues will be positive and based on what has gone well in the interview, and that any suggestions for improvement will be made in a constructive way. Thus when a participant plays the part of the interview that they were least happy with, rather than criticism of poor practice, they should expect that colleagues will generate some solutions as to how the tape could be improved with the value of hindsight.

If participants have agreed to interview an actual patient between the introductory session and the following week, they will need to have time to read the written briefing notes and to ask any questions. This is important so that everyone goes away with a very clear idea of the task in hand. The tutor should expect, even with very careful groundwork, that in the period between contracting to make the tape and making it, at least one participant will be on the phone expressing some difficulties. If all else fails and that particular participant cannot get a patient or relative for whatever reason, it could be suggested that they ask a partner or friend to take the role of a patient so that they can do the nearest equivalent to a simulated interview. The alternative is to have one or two simulated patients available at the beginning of the next session for those people who have been unable to make a tape in their own time.

THE FEEDBACK SESSION

It is useful to start the feedback session by asking participants to share their experiences and feelings about interviewing the patient on their audio-tape. If simulated patients have been used, this is often the point at which the participants will ask, 'Was it a real patient?' The tutor might feel it useful to differentiate between the simulated patient who has had a real experience and an actor, who is someone who has had a brief script of what is expected of them. In using simulated patients, the participants are often very impressed with the reality of the interview and the feelings of the 'patient'. This is because simulators really do appear to relive what it was like when they were coming to grips with a fear-provoking diagnosis, an uncertain future and perhaps frightening treatment. Other issues raised include the fear that tape-recording interviews for the participant's benefit is somehow unfair or even harmful to the patient. General discussion of this kind sets the scene for the feedback on the actual interactions made by the group.

After this introductory time, the tutor should negotiate with the group about how the session will take place and set out some of the agreements made when the contract was set and the way in which the tutor will facilitate. The tutor may start this part of the session by saying:

> 'Now, can I be reminded which three of you are going to play parts of your tape today ... so it was John, Mary and Sam, OK? Now, you remember from last week that what we want you to do is to first of all give us a thumbnail sketch of the patient you saw and then play the part of your tape that you felt most pleased about. We will then give you some feedback and share what was good before I ask for any suggestions on how it could be even better. After that I will ask you to play part of the tape where you are not so pleased. Maybe you picked up a problem and you weren't sure what to do with it, but that's entirely your choice. What I will expect the rest of you to do is to generate some ideas as to how, with the wonder of hindsight, that particular part of the interview could have been improved.

'May I remind you that either the person who is playing the tape or myself can stop it at any time. The reason for stopping it will normally be a particular point that needs to be discussed or it could be, from my point of view, a teaching point where something especially good has happened. I may also ask questions of the group in terms of what you predict is going to happen following a particular sequence. The player may wish to stop at any point, maybe to raise issues or for similar reasons to those I've given for myself. Right, now have you decided who's going first? Mary – OK. Mary, do you want to tell us something about your patient?'

The first participant to play part of their tape may well be very tense and worried. In giving them a chance to say something about the patient first, they will have a few minutes to gather their wits before they disclose how they sound on an audio-tape and what sort of an interview style they have. The exchange may goes as follows:

Mary:	'This was a patient who'd been newly admitted with diabetes and was needing to be stabilized on insulin. I hadn't talked to her before so I was doing a first assessment.'
Tutor:	'Right, now which part of your tape are you going to play that you're particularly pleased with?'
Mary:	'It's the first part right from the beginning because I'm not very pleased with quite a lot of this tape, but I do think that I introduce myself and put her at ease and get her talking about how she'd found out about what was going on quite well, particularly since she was surprised that she had to come into hospital to be stabilized, and I think I dealt with that quite well.'
Tutor:	'OK, let's play that part and see how it goes, and don't forget I may stop it before you ask to stop it. If any member of the group wants to stop it, you'll have to give clear signals and then a very clear reason as to why you wanted to stop it at that point.'

The first part of the tape is played with as many stops as seems to be required and at each stop the group is asked to make positive comments on what they have heard and, only when positive comment has been exhausted, to make some constructive suggestions if applicable for an improved performance. The tutor will then ask the participant to play a part of the tape with which they are less happy, and this might go as follows:

Mary:	'I'm playing you this bit because you'll hear that the patient became really upset and I didn't know what to do with it (starts the tape at the new place).'
Patient:	'Life's never going to be the same, is it nurse?'

Nurse: 'What do you mean by that?'
Patient: (Beginning to weep.) 'Well, I'll be different from everybody else. For the rest of my life I won't be able to eat or drink or do anything the same as I am now. All the time I'll have to start thinking about injections and measuring food and worrying about what's in drink (heavy weeping).'

Mary may stop the tape at this point and the tutor may ask:

'Can you tell me what was so difficult for you about that particular sequence, Mary?'

Mary: 'Well, I didn't know what to say. After all, to a certain extent she's right, isn't she? Her whole life is going to change. I just felt so sorry for her.'
Tutor: 'Well, I'm going to turn this one over to the group now. You'll all have heard from the first part of Mary's tape that she was doing an excellent job in helping this patient disclose her knowledge of the disease and her reactions and feelings about becoming a diabetic. But in spite of all this, Mary has been faced with a patient who begins to react with tears and distress. I wonder if any of you can suggest how Mary might handle that particular problem of a patient who begins weeping and seems to be totally upset and demoralized.'

The group can then be encouraged to look at ways of handling emotion and it is possible that other teaching can be recalled to remind the group how one handles emotional reactions. However, the tutor should intervene with solutions or potential solutions only when the group has exhausted its own repertoire. This will give value to the opinions of the group and help to encourage them to work with each other on both positive feedback and constructive suggestions that are well thought out.

Once the first feedback has been given and the group begins to see that it is a positive experience, the next participant may not feel quite so nervous. But each participant should be given time and space to describe their patient, why they chose them and why they are playing particular parts of the tape to the rest of the group. The tutor who is taking the role of facilitator also needs to check the group, as in a role play session, to make sure that members of the group are not becoming distressed or triggered by what they are hearing on the audio-tape.

CONCLUDING THE SESSION

At the end of the session the tutor should thank those people who put themselves on the line on the first feedback session, saying something along the lines of:

'Well, I want to thank the three of you very much for taking the first session of audio feedback. We've heard some really good material this afternoon, three very well chosen patients, and we've also generated a lot of discussion on how to handle difficult parts of an assessment interview. Can I just clarify which three of you going to bring your tapes for next week's session and ask you to agree among yourselves the order in which you present, and remember it will be just the same as this week.

'I will ask for a thumbnail sketch of the patient that you interviewed and we'll then need to have you describe the part you're most pleased with and play that to us, and the part that you are least pleased with and play that to us. You'll have seen from this afternoon that the part that you play need only be a few minutes long to generate quite a lot of very useful discussion. I've enjoyed this session, I hope you found it useful too. See you all next week. Thank you.'

POTENTIAL DIFFICULTIES

It will have been seen that careful planning and adequate negotiation with the group should reduce the number of difficulties of gaining co-operation from all the group members. However, difficulties can occur and it is worth thinking of the sort of problems that might be encountered. These will depend largely on who the group members are and why they are there.

If the participants are attending a workshop because they are highly motivated to improve their skills, they are far more likely to be co-operative than if the group is learning about communication as part of the prescribed course to which they are obliged to attend. Similarly, with the individual who has been sent on a course rather than having the freedom to choose whether that course was the one that they wished to attend. These participants may well resist exposing any deficits in their skills.

In any group it is normally only one or perhaps two members who cause difficulties in terms of their co-operation. The reasons for their difficulties tend to follow a fairly regular pattern.

No suitable patient

The most common alibi for not bringing an audio-tape to a session is that there were no patients during the previous week or the time allowed that were suitable to be interviewed. This is difficult to dispute, though perhaps also difficult to believe, but rather than confront the participant and throw doubt on their assertion, it is preferable to make some other arrangements so that they can in fact do an interview as described on page 55 prior to the start of the next session. If the course or workshop is being held in or very near to a hospital or hospice, it may be possible to make arrangements on one of the wards for participants to go there to interview a patient between one session and the next. Few participants are totally resistant to interviewing but some may be so nervous that they continue to put if off until they are actually faced with a patient with a tape recorder in their hand in a situation that has been arranged by the tutor. This problem does not occur when simulators are used, and very few participants refuse to carry out the interview.

Unsuitable interviewee

When interviewing patients, even with a written handout on the exact nature of the task, it occasionally occurs that a participant will bring along a tape recording of a totally unsuitable interview. Because of the nature of the feedback session, the tutor would not normally have heard any part of the audio-tape prior to the session and may be faced with having part of an interview played that simply does not conform to the aims of the particular session. Hopefully, this will be picked up when the participant describes the patient that she interviewed. For example:

Tutor: 'Sam, you were the last one in this session. I wonder if you'd like to tell us something about your patient, and then, as you've seen, play the part of your tape that you are most pleased with.'

Sam: 'Er, well, actually I didn't interview a patient, I interviewed a relative.'

Tutor: 'Can you tell me why you did that, Sam?'

Sam: 'Well, the thing was there wasn't a suitable patient. The patients on our ward are all quite ill and I didn't think it was fair, so what I did was to interview a relative.'

Tutor: 'Can you tell us something about that relative?'

Sam: 'Oh yes, it was a relative who was coming to pick the patient up for discharge, so the whole interview was to do with the discharge procedure and arrangements for follow-up.'

Tutor: 'Let me stop you there, Sam. I can see from what you're saying that you have a very good reason for not interviewing a patient but the purpose of this session is to look at assessment techniques and I don't really think that the discharge procedure would fit into that. What do you think?'

Sam: 'Well, no I suppose not. Sorry, yeah, I knew that wasn't the best thing to do but I was stuck. It was yesterday, I knew the session was today and I simply didn't know quite what was going to occur.'

Tutor: 'Well look, let's leave it there. We've got two more sessions
            on feedback and that gives you time to actually interview a
            patient using the written guidelines you've got, but of
            course that does leave us with a little time this afternoon. I
            wonder has anyone else got their tape with them, even
            though they weren't expecting to have feedback today?'

After this sort of exchange there is almost always someone who has their
tape with them who will step into the breach and this should be properly
acknowledged. At the end of such a session it is worth having a private
word with Sam to check out that there are not any real problems in
making the sort of tape that has been agreed by the whole group.

The alternative is to let Sam play part of his 'discharge procedure with
a relative' tape. The reasons for this not being the best idea is that it can
irritate the whole group to have something different brought into a
session that had been clearly prescribed and agreed by the group. If
Sam's situation is handled sensitively, hopefully with a little humour, he
will not come out of the situation feeling silly but if he *does* play his tape
and the group *does* get annoyed, that could be more damaging to him in
the long run.

No time

Not having time to fulfil a task between one session and the next is
another reasonably common alibi. 'We've just been so busy, two staff
have been off sick ...' are well known reasons given for not making an
audio-tape. Again, this is a situation where a tutor will probably gain
more insight if he or she has a word with the participant during the
coffee or lunch break to see if there are any underlying reasons why the
interview has not been undertaken. If it genuinely is that the ward has
been in chaos for the last week, then this might be another situation
where the tutor will arrange for a patient, a time and the wherewithal to
record an interview based on that individual's own work area.

Too nervous

Some participants really are quite frightened of audio-recording an interview with a patient. Such nervousness needs to be explored and often is
found to be due to a previous poor experience, either in role play or in
some other interactive situation that causes the participant to feel that
they cannot make themselves vulnerable enough to allow colleagues to
hear how they interview a patient. This is a situation that calls for
particularly sensitive handling and usually, if the cause of the
nervousness is explored and understood, the participant may well be
persuaded to 'have a go' no matter what.

Occasionally, students are nervous because they feel that they themselves are so unskilled that they could not face their colleagues hearing the tape. In this situation it does sometimes help if the tutor offers to pre-hear the audio-tape before the session and helps the participant to pick out those areas that are worth positive feedback and to pick out an area for discussion on improvement that is not too contentious. Almost inevitably at such a preview, the tutor will find that the student is no better or worse than anyone else in the group, but is far harder on themselves in terms of the standards that they expect.

It will be seen from this that since there is always a risk that somebody who is due to have audio-feedback may not bring a tape with them, some contingency plans may be useful. In negotiating with the group for who is going to present next week, it would help if a fourth person was prepared to be a stand-in. This could be negotiated as follows:

'We've agreed who is going to have audio feedback on their tapes next week but I think we have to face the fact that sometimes things get in the way and people don't always arrive, and there is a lot of 'flu around at the moment, for example. So I think it would be quite sensible to have somebody else who has hasn't had feedback yet, to agree to be a standby next week so that if we do have any gaps there's somebody there ready to step in. I wonder if anybody would be prepared to do that. I know it means bringing your tape two weeks running but it's better than having a gap which might be quite difficult to fill. Right, thanks very much Charles, that's really kind of you. OK.'

If communication skills as a subject is going through a whole course, which means that after the first module of however many weeks, the students may come back at a following stage in their course, it is worth asking them to save their initial audio-tapes. When they come in for the next module that includes communication skills, they can be asked to make a new audio-tapes and comparisons can be made to help them see how they have advanced and which areas they still need to work on. The only difficulty with this is for those individuals who do not seem to have improved their communication skills. Even here, it is usually possible to find some positives before tackling the areas where extra work needs to be done.

Overall, audio feedback is an enjoyable and pleasant teaching method once participants have been reassured both by negotiation and, hopefully, the first session that this type of learning can be a very positive experience. It does require great sensitivity on the part of the teacher, allied with a total belief that everyone in the group will participate.

SUMMARY

In this chapter audio feedback as a teaching method has been considered both in terms of interviews with participants' patients on their own wards and interviews made while on the course using simulated patients. The importance of planning has been considered, along with group size, methods of briefing and the need to contract with the group to gain co-operation. Handling a feedback session has also been considered along with potential difficulties with individuals who, for one reason or another, may not make an audio-tape of their interactions. Suggestions have been given as to how to deal with potential problems of non-co-operation.

REFERENCES

Faulkner, A. (1992) The evaluation of training programmes for communication skills in palliative care. *Journal of Cancer Care*, **1**(2), 75–8.
Faulkner, A. and Maguire, P. (1983) Teaching ward nurses to monitor cancer patients. *Clinical Oncology*, **10**, 383–9.
Maguire, P., Faulkner, A. and Fairbairn, S. (1989) *Training Community Nurses to Assess and Monitor Patients with Cancer*. Report to the Cancer Research Campaign, London.

CHAPTER SIX

The discussion session

Discussion sessions can be a dynamic teaching method for topics which do not require a formal lecture and are not suitable for role play, audio feedback or, indeed, video demonstration. There are many advantages to using this teaching method.

1. Discussion uses the expertise within the group and is particularly useful when the group may be of mixed disciplines or of the same disciplines but from different specialties or of different grades. Group members participating in the discussion will feel that their knowledge and experience is being valued by the whole group.
2. Discussion promotes sharing in a relatively safe environment and may help participants to appreciate different perspectives to the same problem.
3. Discussion sessions can help participants to generalize solutions from one problem to another and realize that strategies are also generalizable. There may also be an element of discovery learning present in a discussion session.

SUBJECT CHOICE

The subjects of a discussion session should be those where there is room for debate. If the course/workshop is based on an agenda set by the participants, suitable topics may be negotiated with the group. In a pre-planned programme, discussion sessions can be included. Problem areas that are very useful for discussion include those where there are:

- family difficulties;
- team problems;
- ethical dilemmas;
- spiritual issues;
- contentious issues.

It will be seen from the above that discussion sessions do not necessarily end with a consensus. What they do is to encourage debate and help participants to accept that there are differing views on the best solutions to a number of problems. This movement from 'right versus wrong' to shades of agreement and perhaps consensus encourage participants to gain insights into other's perspectives.

In using discussion as a teaching method, the facilitator must be very careful not to influence the debate and to have as open a view as possible, especially when the discussion is on topics where there may be no right or wrong answers.

PLANNING THE SESSION

When planning the session, the size of the group is extremely important. If there are less than 20 participants in a group then the leader may decide to have discussion with the whole group on the topic of choice. Alternatively, the group may be split into two smaller groups and each group will discuss the topic and then feed back to the larger group. If this method is chosen then a decision has to be made as to whether the small groups will work with a leader or without.

Depending on the subject under debate, having one of the tutors as a leader to a group of 10 or indeed to the whole group of 20 can be an advantage because this will allow some control in terms of members of the group who have strong opinions versus others who may not readily articulate their views. Alternatively, it can be argued that if a tutor is with the group during a discussion session it may inhibit participation.

It is possible to plan a discussion session with a large group of 50 or more providing that there are enough rooms to split that group into small subgroups. Again, with this method of teaching a decision has to be made on whether outside group leaders are required or whether the group can appoint its own leader and reporter. Some of the above decisions may be coloured by the format of the course or workshop in which discussion is one of the teaching methods. For example, on a study day where participants will not have met each other before and may not be meeting each other again, a facilitator is necessary to encourage participation and sharing in what may seem to be a difficult situation until group members learn a little about each other.

If discussion as a teaching method is used in a workshop or as part of an ongoing course on effective interaction, then both the topic and the timing of the discussion will help to set the decision as to whether a leader is required. As seen in Chapter 12, small groups with a facilitator who is a member of the group work very well when setting an agenda. In that instance the agenda is to do with the individual and the professional 'luggage' that they have brought to the course or workshop.

Such an exercise, discussing common problems, can build trust to a level where subsequently a discussion group can consider far more contentious areas than the problems that participants have brought with them. These include ethical dilemmas, spiritual issues and other issues which require people to share their views and project their ideas for solution to particular problems.

If a discussion session is planned that includes a relatively large group, that is, 50 or more, the time will have to be carefully allotted to allow: (1) enough time for debate; and (2) enough time for feedback and sharing in the large group if this is seen to be appropriate.

If the group is appointing its own leader, then there has to be clear ground rules as to how they report back. It may be that each group is asked to summarize their discussion into five main points that have emerged. If the group is not divided into smaller groups, the course tutor or a colleague can build up the summary during the session using a flip chart.

If groups are to work on their own, then in planning the session, the facilitator has to decide whether he/she will 'float' or whether to leave the groups entirely on their own to fulfil the task in hand. The topic under discussion may affect the decision but overall, once a group has started working, they usually work best if there are no interruptions from outside. This requires trust on the tutor's part and clear thinking in advance as to the possible problems that might arise in discussing a particular subject. As a rule of thumb, the more contentious the issue the more appropriate it is for a tutor/facilitator to run the group discussion.

Once a discussion topic is set it is often useful to have a number of questions ready to generate discussion if participants in the group are not eager to start a debate. It might be, for example, that the discussion topic is dealing with family problems when a patient is in hospital. If this topic comes from an agenda that has been set then there will have been an example of family problems identified. The following problem was identified as an agenda item on a Help the Hospice Workshop:

Joseph: 'I sometimes think that when a patient is in the hospice the family is ganging up against me.'
Tutor: 'Can you give me an example of that, Joe?'
Joseph: 'Yes. We had this lady admitted for respite care and we put her in a single room. It's got a nice balcony with lovely views, and I went along to do the first assessment, to see how she was settling in and all her family were there and I felt...I felt almost like an intruder.'

An opening question to start debate on family issues, given the above example, might be, 'Joe, you gave us this problem, I wonder if you can share with the group what it was that made you feel like an intruder.' Another more general question to the whole group might be, 'How many of the rest of you have had this sort of experience of being outnumbered by the family?' This second question will encourage group members to feel free to share their experiences of dealing with a whole family rather than an individual patient. Two or three of these questions ready at hand will help most group discussions to get started with little difficulty, particularly if the discussion topic is centred around an area of clinical practice that is pertinent to the group.

THE SESSION

In opening a discussion session it is important to make clear the purpose of the session and what is expected from the participants. Given Joseph's problem, the following introduction might be made.

Tutor: 'We are going to discuss family issues this afternoon and I though we'd start with the problem that Joe brought up as an agenda item yesterday morning. Joe, I wonder if you could briefly remind us of the main problem.'

Joseph: 'Well, it was this patient that we had put in a single room ...all her family were around her and I went to do an assessment, actually not knowing they were there, and I just felt like an intruder.'

Tutor: 'Right. What I want to do is to look at Joe's problem and I am going to ask you all to think about whether you have had a similar problem and then we'll discuss how one sets about handling a family who may possibly be quite tense and upset and worried.'

As participants in the group share their problems of dealing with whole families who sometimes may be loathe to leave the patient alone with a health professional, the facilitator must keep clearly in their mind the purpose of the session. Joe's problem, for example, brings up many issues. It brings up the issue of the patient's personal space, and the family's feelings about their rights in their loved one's illness. In this situation it can be forgotten that the problem put forward by Joe was more to do with his feelings of inadequacy in the face of a tight-knit family unit. In order to help Joe with his problem, other related issues will emerge, but it is important not to lose sight of the focus of the discussion.

Participants' contribution to the discussion may not always be in line with the objectives of the session, nor yet may solutions offered be practical or, indeed, possible. The risk here is that the participant who has made an inappropriate suggestion needs nevertheless to feel that there is some value in the contribution even if it is not the best option. This is illustrated below.

1. Tutor: 'It seems that Joe is not alone in having this problem of feeling like an intruder when a family are all around the bed. Can anyone suggest what options Joe has for finding a solution to this dilemma?'

	Suzie:	'He could ask the family to go...he could tell them that he is a busy doctor and has to do the basic assessment and tell them to come back another time.'
	Tutor:	'That's just going to put their back up...you can't do that. Has anybody got a better suggestion than that?'
2.	Tutor:	'It seems that Joe is not alone in having this problem of feeling like an intruder when a family are all around the bed. Can anyone suggest what options Joe has for finding a solution to this dilemma?'
	Suzie:	'He could ask the family to go...he could tell them that he is a busy doctor and has to do the basic assessment and tell them to come back another time.'
	Tutor:	'Well, he could ask them to leave but I wonder can anyone in the group see a problem with this approach?'
	Penny:	'Isn't it going to upset them a bit...you said yourself that they were likely to be tense and upset...maybe he could put off the assessment until later and while he is in the room with the whole family introduce himself to them.'

In the first example, the tutor dismissed turning the family out as an option in a way that would leave Suzie feeling perhaps silly but also perhaps a little damaged that her suggestion was thrown out rather roughly. In the second example, the tutor is accepting that this is one option and is leaving it to the group to generate ideas as to why it may not be the best way forward. This second approach is much more sensitive and is likely to leave Suzie able to see for herself that although one *can* ask a family to go, it is not always the best or most appropriate action to take. This ability to use all suggestions in a positive way encourages participants to offer their thoughts on how to solve often quite difficult problems. It also encourages the group to offer alternatives in a sensitive way. This part of discussion is very similar to the generating of solutions that occurs in role play.

Many discussions are very concerned with feelings. Joe's problem, for example, is very much to do with how he feels when he is confronted by a family. His feelings of being an intruder have prevented him from handling the situation as well as he would like. This also holds true on discussions of problems within the interdisciplinary team and, certainly in both ethical and spiritual issues, there is the potential for the expression of feelings. Sometimes within a discussion it is possible to stop and concentrate on those feelings by asking members of the group to mime how they are feeling in a certain situation. This is often called sculpting but in this book it will not be considered as a separate teaching method, but rather as an exercise that can be used within a discussion and which may not last for very long. It has a number of advantages:

1. It concentrates a discussion for a limited period of time on feelings above all else;
2. It puts members of the group into the skin of another individual for a short time so that they can begin to appreciate the feelings of that other individual;
3. It allows the actors in the exercise to each give their perspective of what is happening;
4. It can, but does not always, generate possible solutions to a specific problem.

A SCULPTING EXERCISE

In a sculpting exercise the individual who offered the problem is asked to select the major players in the problem as follows:

Tutor:	'Joe, I wonder if we could take a little time to sculpt your problem. Can you choose people out of the group to make up the key players?'
Joe:	'Well, yes all right...Mary, would you be the patient?'
Tutor:	'Mary, can you come and stand in the circle?'
Joe:	'Harry, could you be Mary's husband?'
Tutor:	'Harry, could you come into the circle? Joe, would you put Harry where you think he belongs in terms of the problem you described to us?'
Joe:	'Yes...Harry, could you go and stand very close to Mary... and Anne, could you be her daughter?'
Tutor:	'Anne, can you join this family unit...where do you want her, Joe?'
Joe:	'If she could come the other side of Mary, and I need just one more...Hannah, could you be the other daughter and could you be sort of in front of them...not quite so close but still quite close?'
Tutor:	'Thank you, Joe, but have you forgotten to choose someone who will take on your role?'
Joe:	'Oh...John, would you do that?'
John:	'Yes, I don't mind...where do you want me?'
Joe:	'Over here, as if you are in the doorway and the family is over there.'

Setting up the sculpt in this way allows Joe to demonstrate with other members of the group just how he saw the family and it becomes obvious from the way he sets them out (Figure 6.1) that to him the family were tightly linked, with him at a considerable distance from the rest of them.

(A)

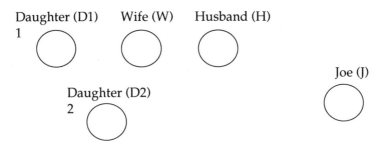

Positions in original scenario (problem)

(B)

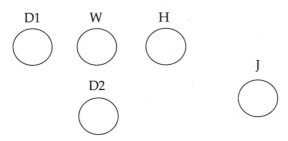

Positions of players' choice (towards solution)

Figure 6.1 Changing positions in a sculpting exercise.

The tutor then asks each member of the group how they feel in their situation. It might go as follows:

Tutor: 'You are all in the positions that Joe has put you in and I want you to think yourself into who you are. I'm going to ask you first...Mary, as the patient, how do you feel where you are at the moment?'

Mary: 'I feel very protected...it's good to have my family so close round me when underneath I am a bit frightened.'

Tutor: 'What are you frightened of?'

Mary: 'Well, I can see the doctor over there and I'm frightened of what he's going to say to me, but I don't feel quite so frightened because my family are all here.'

Tutor:	'Harry, as the husband, can I ask you how you're feeling where you are?'
Harry:	'Well, I just want to look after Mary...after all, it can't be very good for her and I feel that I'm here to protect her.'
Tutor:	'Are you feeling anything else?'
Harry:	'Well, I'm feeling glad that she's got this area to herself so that we can be here when she needs us.'
Tutor:	'And how do you feel about the doctor?'
Harry:	'Well, he doesn't seem to know what he's doing...he's just stood in the doorway looking a bit uncertain...I do hope that he is more effective than he looks because I want Mary to be in safe hands.'
Tutor:	'Anne, as a daughter, how do you feel?'
Anne:	'I feel a bit embarrassed really...I mean, all right Mary is in the bed...she's the patient and I'm here as her daughter but I can't do anything...there's a doctor in the doorway...I'd like to talk to him...I'd like to ask him what's going to happen and he's not coming in he's just stood there.'
Hannah:	'I feel a bit like that too, in fact I feel a bit of a prune stood here not quite so much with the others...I wonder if in fact Anne is closer to the mother than I am...I'm not sure of my position here at all.'
Tutor:	'We'll come back to that, but John...you're the doctor ...how do you feel?'
John:	'Well, it may be because of what Joe has told us but I do feel as if I can't go into that family because they don't seem to need me at the moment...I'm here to help...I would have expected them to be very welcoming and I don't quite know how to break into their circle.'
Tutor:	'Right, well you have all said something about the way you feel in the position that you have been put in. What I want you to do now, each of you, is to move to where you would like to be...if it's where you are now that's OK... don't move...but if any of you want to move then would you do it now.'

This second part of the exercise is designed to see what will happen when individuals are given the freedom to move out of the area they have been put in. It may be that John will try and move towards the family, but if they do not want him, it may be that they will then move much closer to each other. It is important to remember that the tutor will not know what the players are going to do.

   In the sculpt that was actually played out with Joe's problem, what happened was exactly that. John in Joe's role moved closer to the family and the family all moved in much more closely to each other. This move-ment in itself was quite dramatic but even more important was the feelings that each player described when the tutor went back to them. Family members described how they felt threatened in the main by John trying to get closer to them, but John had the insight to see that in fact it was not that the family were not allowing him in, but that, in fact, he was intruding and that the problem was his.

This insight helped Joe enormously, who said, 'Well, yes, that's right. I suppose for them that room became their space and then I had to seek permission to enter it if they were all there.' Asked what he would do if he could re-run his own problem with the family, he said, 'Well, it might upset my work schedule but I think I would just leave them, given that they are all coming to grips with the patient's admission, and I would go back and see the patient later on when she had settled down and her family had gone home.'

All sculpts do not work out as well as that but if they are carefully set up and each player is given the right to say exactly how they feel, there can be enormous value in terms of gaining insight into how different individuals feel in a particular situation. The reality value can be enhanced if the players are not called by their own names once they have been put into the sculpt but are called by who they are portraying. For example, the tutor would not say, 'Mary, how do you feel there?' but would say, 'I want to ask the patient...how do you feel?' or 'I want to ask the patient's husband...how are you feeling?' This reminds everybody who the players are portraying.

In exercises like this it is interesting that individuals are far more ready to take part than they often are in role play. This may be because they are assured that they will not be expected to speak when they are in role but to simply do what feels right and then describe to the group what taking that action made them feel. The other interesting point is that almost all groups who take part in this type of exercise during a discussion period describe the feelings as very potent. This means that the tutor has a responsibility to check up that there are no residual feelings of grief or emotion following the session. In fact, the discussion that follows a sculpting exercise usually has the effect of debriefing the players.

In planning a discussion session it is not always possible to decide when or what will be sculpted. This exercise works best if it can be used spontaneously when the situation appears to merit it. That may not sound very constructive advice for a teacher and, indeed, there is no reason why sculpts should not be planned. This is a matter of individual choice. The ability to use the exercise spontaneously is much easier when the facilitator feels fairly secure in the material that he/she is using and asking people to discuss.

POTENTIAL PROBLEMS

The major problems in a discussion group are at two ends of the same continuum. One represents the individual who wants to talk all the time and the other is the individual who does not appear to want to contribute at all. Both require sensitive handling by the tutor and will be considered in Chapter 8. In sculpting exercises there is a risk of individuals who do not wish to participate, but this seems to be much less of a problem than in role play, which can seem a more threatening exercise.

SUMMARIZING THE SESSION

Full group with facilitator

If the facilitator has the whole group of 16 to 20 participants for a discussion period then it is possible, as points are made that are important to the discussion, to write them up on a flip chart or a board in order to build a summary of the session. The difficulty with this is that, in a group discussion, points are not always brought out in the order that the facilitator would require in terms of the summary. This can be remedied at the end of the session by coming back to the flip chart and saying:

> 'We have a lot of important points up here. Let me summarize them in what I think is the order of importance. Obviously, I am open to any suggestions from the group so if you don't agree with the priority in which I am putting them, please let me know.'

Priorities are not always important, of course, and much depends on the discussion as to what are seen to be key points. These should relate to the original questions that were posed in the planning of the discussion group.

Small groups with no facilitator

When small groups reconvene, each bringing several points to summarize their discussions, the facilitator needs to take the points from the first group reporter and then as other groups report, build up a picture from the group. In this instance one would expect quite a lot of overlap in terms of points that have been raised. If, for example, the group has been discussing spiritual issues, there will be common elements from each of the groups, but there will also be highly individual elements coming out which will reflect the composition of each of the smaller groups and the unique contribution that each member of the group has given to the discussion.

No matter whether the discussion has taken part in smaller or larger groups, it is important that the session is concluded with a summary of the discussion so that individuals have the whole discussion put into some sort of context for them.

The facilitator can in fact include the whole group in this exercise. To return to Joe's problem, it may be that at the end of the session the facilitator has a number of points on the flip chart to do with families and how they feel in times of crisis, and also points about health professionals and their role in working with families. In Joe's case, it can be shown how a health professional may feel when confronted by a frightened family. The facilitator might then say, 'We have quite a lot of points on the board about family issues, and the role of the health professional with the family, as well as with the individual patient. I wonder if anyone would like to start looking at these points and putting them in any sort of order of importance.'

By making this sort of offer to the group, everyone feels involved in the whole experience, including summarizing at the end. This will take longer than if the tutor alone is going to summarize, and adequate time should be built into the planning of the session.

SUMMARY

In this chapter, discussion has been considered as a teaching method to discuss problems and difficulties in effective interaction that are not really suitable for other teaching methods such as role play, audio feedback or video discussion. It has been seen that discussion uses the experience within the group and promotes sharing. It also fosters generalization and discovery learning.

To be effective, discussion sessions have to be planned carefully in terms of subject choice, group format, numbers and the objectives of the session. In the session itself, participants need to be encouraged to take part and this can be effected by positively using all contributions even if they cannot be accepted as a best option.

Sculpting exercises have been considered as a possibility for using within a discussion session and, finally, the need to summarize a discussion session has been discussed.

PART TWO

Problems, Costs and Measurement

CHAPTER SEVEN

Potential difficulties

With careful planning and execution, it is possible to run a course or workshop on effective interaction with patients with few difficulties. The priority will be that the group will work as a cohesive whole to improve and develop their skills, knowledge and attitudes towards effective interaction. There are, however, potential difficulties to which a tutor needs to be alert so that should any of them arise, prompt action can be taken and further difficulties avoided. Some of these problems, such as triggering, can be caused because of the interactive nature of the work. Others can occur in any group no matter what the subject to be taught or how it is being taught, such as a participant who is disruptive or a constant late arriver.

If difficulties do arise within a group, the tutor should stay as calm as possible and not become defensive, no matter how much he/she is challenged. Very often a quiet approach will be much more effective than confrontation. Below, some of the common difficulties are considered with suggestions for dealing with them.

PERSONAL VERSUS PROFESSIONAL ISSUES

In other chapters, the advantages of teaching effective interactive skills based on clinical problems of the group are extolled. The other side of that coin is that in any teaching that asks for experiential material, there is a risk that some participants may wish to bring up issues that are more personal than professional. Such participants will see a workshop or a course as a vehicle for working through their own problems even when the tutor has made it clear when briefing the group that their agenda should be based on professional problems. This is not always a deliberate attempt to bring in personal issues, but what comes to mind when thinking of clinical problems may be influenced by unconscious worries on a personal front. It can be seen in Chapter 12 that in an agenda-setting session the problems identified are screened by the tutor to check exactly where they come from and where they apply. In Chapter 10 the importance of screening out a problem that is too close to home is also shown.

No matter the situation, whether setting an agenda, setting up a role play or, indeed, giving a formal or semi-formal lecture on a difficult area such as bereavement, the tutor is dependent on participants' honesty. It is important to point this out to group members and also to make absolutely clear that the course or workshop has the aim of improving interactive skills and is not there for a cathartic experience.

This approach may appear to be over-careful in terms of the stress put on the aims of the course, the nature of the agenda to which the group will work and the care for the members of the group. The rationale for such stress both at the beginning and throughout the course is based on the experience that if personal issues are brought into the forum, then difficulties will ensue. This applies not only to the participant who wants to share his on her problems, but for the group as a whole, which may not be able to deal with the information given. The individual, if he or she is allowed to disclose personal problems, may disclose too much and then be very embarrassed at meeting the group and working with them later on. The group members, too, may be very embarrassed and may perhaps even take sides on what is an appropriate answer. What happens then is that, instead of a session that is helping to improve skills in a professional setting, group members will find themselves moving into therapeutic mode. This is unacceptable unless the whole group has agreed to use the time in such a way, and the tutor has the necessary skills to handle the session.

The following is an example of what might happen in a situation where the professional problem is overshadowed by a personal one. Sally had identified an agenda item on anger. She gave a scenario where an elderly lady was in hospital and her daughter was very dissatisfied with the care being given. Sally offered to role play the patient and, when screened, assured the tutor that this was not too close to home in any way. Half way through the role play, Sally burst into tears and started telling the group about her dying mother who she felt very guilty about because she could not visit as often as she would like to. When she did visit, she was never satisfied with what was going on.

At this point the tutor stopped Sally and said, 'It looks as if the problem that you gave us was in fact very closely linked to a personal problem. You may not have realized this but I can see you're upset and I think we should stop this role play now. Would you like to say any more to the group or would you rather we left it until later?' Sally decided to leave it until later when she was able to talk through with the tutor the nature of her problem. As a result she contracted to go to the hospital and, as calmly as she could, tell them how unhappy she was.

It could be argued that this problem could have been aired in front of the whole group. The rationale here for making it less public is linked with the fact that Sally has to work with the group after such disclosures and should not be left to feel that she has said too much to too many.

If the link between the material being used in the class is linked unconsciously with a personal problem of a student, then triggering may occur.

TRIGGERING

One of the difficulties of using interactive teaching methods is that the tutor, when planning the course and the material to be covered, cannot know what personal 'luggage' each participant brings with them. What can be certain is that no-one will arrive for any session in neutral. What is also important to realize is that individuals who are working on such a course will not necessarily know what sort of material might trigger them, for if someone has had something very difficult or unpleasant happen to them in the past, they may well have 'put the lid on' that experience and closed their minds to it. What will trigger such a memory is often something quite small, and although it does not happen very often, the tutor needs to be alert to the fact that triggering is possible when handling difficult material such as clinical problems, bereavement and other areas involving deep emotions.

In obvious areas such as sessions on bereavement, the tutor can screen for anyone who may find it difficult by saying, for example, 'This next session on bereavement is likely to be quite heavy. If any of you have been bereaved in the recent past and feel that this would be too painful, then please feel free to go to the library and I'll give you a handout later on the material covered.' In fact, such an offer is seldom taken up since most participants feel that they can deal with whatever comes to them. Indeed, triggering often occurs in a totally unexpected way, as follows:

Jane, an experienced nurse, was on a course and agreed to role play a 'confronting colleagues' session where she, in fact, would be the difficult colleague and someone else from the group would confront her with undesirable behaviour. Jane herself had given the problem as an agenda item and had explained that she was having difficulty with her manager who would not understand the need for more resources in her particular area. She had agreed to play the role of the recalcitrant manager because she knew the sort of responses that the manager had given.

In this instance, the colleague confronting Jane was quite assertive and before the tutor could stop the role play because she could see that the confronting colleague was getting aggressive, Jane suddenly burst into tears and then ran from room a few seconds later. The tutor asked if someone in the group would go and see if Jane was all right and she went on with the session. At the coffee break she found Jane and talked to her.

Jane subsequently described an incident when her first marriage had broken up, and relayed with absolute clarity the situation she was in when she had felt totally helpless in the face of her husband's infidelity. The colleague who had been confronting her (very successfully) had rekindled that feeling of helplessness in Jane and, in sitting there, not knowing what to say as the recalcitrant manager, she suddenly was transformed back to the last time that she had felt so helpless. This had triggered all the grief about the loss of her marriage that she had shut away at the time that it had happened. She described how everyone had said how wonderfully she had coped at the time, and admitted that her first marriage had not been in her mind in any way when she agreed to the role play. The two items were totally unconnected as far as she was concerned.

It is argued here that if a participant becomes triggered by the events happening around them, that the tutor's place is with the group and that a group member should go to talk to the person who has left the room. If the person does not leave the room but sits obviously very upset, then the tutor should ask her gently if she would like to leave. It is then the participant's choice whether to stay in the room or whether to leave it. In either event the tutor, again, should explore the problem with the participant's permission during a coffee break, and never assume that if someone says, 'I'm OK', that they really mean it.

Triggering can, however, have a beneficial effect as well, though this is more rarely seen. In a recent session entitled 'Child of a dying parent' (Help the Hospices) a young man became very distressed when the section on the angry adolescent was shown. The tutor asked him if he would like to leave and he said he did not want to leave or to talk. He appeared to settle down and accept the rest of the session without any problems.

Over a coffee break the tutor asked the young man if he would like to tell her what the problem had been. He described the death of his mother when he was nine years old and the fact that he had been pushed from pillar to post, from one aunt to another, during his formative years, and then explained that as an adolescent he had been very undisciplined, shoplifting and stealing from his father and committing a number of other 'sins'. He had always blamed himself, from his perspective, for his appalling behaviour and said to the tutor, 'When I saw the video this morning and realized that all that anger was due to the fact that my father had mishandled my mother's death and my involvement in it, then suddenly I was able to let myself off the hook.' Such experiences are very rewarding and also very rare.

Triggering will have an effect on the group for it may be uncomfortable for them to experience someone else's grief. They may turn their attention to the tutor, arguing that either he or she should have gone out after the person who has left the room, or that they should have spent more time being more careful. This need to blame someone for someone else's distress needs to be taken on board by the tutor. If it is talked through, the group will generally realize that the only course of action was the one that was taken.

THE NON-PARTICIPATOR

Any group will include a wide range of personalities, from the extrovert to the very quiet and often non-participating member. It could be argued that if somebody is quiet and does not want to contribute, that is their right. Also, the individual may still be learning and absorbing the content of the session. However, other group members can become quite angry if there is someone who simply does not make any sort of contribution at all. It is therefore quite important to think of how one deals with this without causing the non-participator to feel embarrassed, or the group to feel that they are somehow 'carrying' the non-participator.

As a rule of thumb, there is little point in making an issue of non-participation in the first session or two because different individuals require different amounts of time to feel comfortable enough to take part. However, if the non-participation continues, then the tutor has a choice of exploring what, if any, the problems are and how to deal with them. This can be done in class by directing questions particularly to the participant or out of class where the tutor can ask the participant if there are any problems in terms of contribution.

The problem in asking someone in class a specific question means that they are put on the spot if it concerns something that is totally out of their experience. This can lead to a participant feeling that they are being 'picked on' and made to look small in front of the rest of the group. For this reason alone it may be worth taking to the individual during a coffee or lunch break. The tutor might say something as follows:

Tutor: 'Joan, how are you enjoying the course so far?'
Joan: 'I'm really enjoying it.'
Tutor: 'I wondered, because you're actually very quiet in class.'
Joan: 'I'm actually a very quiet person and the others all seem so clever compared to me.'
Tutor: 'It would be good, though, to hear your opinion some time. I wonder if you could think about that.'

The aim here is to reassure the participant that they are valued as much as other people and that their contribution will be used in a positive way. It also allows the tutor to differentiate between the person who is quiet because that is in their nature and the person who is quiet because they are perhaps hostile to the material being presented or have problems that are getting in the way of their being a full group member. If this latter is the case, then the tutor will need to explore with the participant whether the hostility can be overcome or, indeed, whether this participant should be with the group at all. If the individual is not participating because they are hostile and this is not identified and addressed, then they may well turn into the disruptive participant at a later time.

Sometimes group pressure can deal with non-participation. The tutor may be asking for suggestions for a way forward on a particular topic and one group member may turn to the non-participator and say:

'Jane, you haven't said anything yet. Don't you have any ideas?'

This sort of pressure from the group, if it is handled in a good-humoured way, may well break the deadlock of somebody who is a little nervous of saying what they think. Non-participation is much less likely to occur in an atmosphere where teaching is based on positive feedback and a sense of value is given to each member of the group.

THE OVER-PARTICIPATOR

Just as groups almost always have quiet members, they also have members who seem to want to hold the floor most of the time. What is required here is that the tutor explores to see why this person needs to be always at the forefront, and this must definitely be undertaken away from the main group. The problem is every bit as important as the non-participator because the person who takes over and does not give other people a chance to talk can be even more irritating than someone who does not talk at all. For this reason, group pressure is much more likely to happen sooner rather than later. However, if the group is largely passive and prepared to let someone do all the work, then the tutor will have to step in and control what is happening. The interaction may go as follows:

Tutor: 'Carrie has shared with us that her problem in this role play is that she simply doesn't know how to deal with what seems to be quite justified anger. Has anyone in the group got any ideas?'

John: 'Yes, I don't mind. I'll take over if you like. I don't mind doing this role play; I feel very good about this.'

Tutor: 'Well, no John, that's not what I'm wanting. What I'm asking for are suggestions from all members of the group as to how Carrie can deal with this anger.'

John: 'Well, what she needs to do is to tell the patient that it's OK to be angry.'

Tutor: 'Very good, John. Has anybody else got any ideas?'

John: 'And then...'

Tutor: 'John, I appreciate your input but I'm wondering if other
              people in the group would like to make a contribution too.'

In this sequence, John wanted to take over, but the tutor sensitively
controlled his participation so that he felt valued but was made to
understand that other people had the right to make suggestions. The
important thing here is that the teacher goes back to John so that he does
not feel that he has been closed down forever.

The over-participator does often have a problem and if the tutor talks
to that person they may find that this is somebody who has got a chip on
their shoulder about something in either their personal or professional
lives. In such an instance, the tutor's role is simply to help that
individual to gain some insight into what is happening.

The over-participator can be useful in a group in that if, for example, a
small group is meeting and going to feedback to the larger group, the over-
participator is often a very good choice of person to check that everybody
has a chance to speak up. In this way, they are being invited to take on
more responsibility, but in a way that will control their over-exuberance.
They are also very useful in the first role play or the first audio feedback
session in that often they will jump forward and start the ball rolling.

THE DISRUPTIVE PARTICIPANT

The disruptive participant almost inevitably has a problem. The problem
may or may not be associated with the material that is being covered but
very often there are links. The disruptive participant often shows first as
the non-participator and if this is the case, the quiet hostility is often very
apparent in the way that the participant sits or reacts, even at a non-
verbal level.

The following is an example of a non-participator who was quiet in the
first two sessions and then became disruptive. The material being covered
was 'Talking to AIDS patients and their families' and the particular
problem that had been identified was to do with friction between the
parents of a homosexual AIDS sufferer and the AIDS sufferer's partner.
The tutor suggested a role play between the AIDS sufferer and his
partner, who felt he was being pushed out by the patient's family.

The participant, who up to that time had been very quiet, suddenly
became very vocal about role play and said that he did not feel that role
play was appropriate in sessions to do with AIDS patients. The rest of
the group became very unhappy and the disruptive participant
challenged the tutor as follows:

Guy: 'I do *not* want to role play. I think that it would be damaging
              for everybody and *if* you want role play then you can do it
              without me.'

Tutor: 'Guy, I'm sorry you feel like this. I wonder could you sit down while I negotiate with the rest of the group? We're going to do some role play and I felt we'd agreed to that so what I wanted to do now was to go through the safety rules so that immediately after coffee we could start with the first role play. I wonder how you feel about that in view of Guy's obvious antipathy to the idea?'

Marge: 'Well, why don't you go through the ground rules. I don't mind role playing, I don't know about anybody else.'

Margaret: 'I don't mind either. I don't know what's the matter with you, Guy.'

Guy: 'I've made myself clear.'

Tutor: 'Well, look, let's go through the ground rules for role play, and I have to say now Guy that if you don't want to do the role play, then I suggest you go to the library after coffee.'

During the coffee break the tutor found Guy and asked him if he would come into her office, and then she asked him why he was so angry before the role play had even started. Guy was very quiet and then after careful exploration from the tutor admitted that he was, in fact, a homosexual and that his lover was currently in hospital very sick. He felt that the whole business of AIDS was difficult for him.

The tutor was very puzzled because she did not understand quite why he was on a course which she had been told comprised nurses who had all requested to attend. At this point, Guy admitted that he had been sent on the course by his manager who felt that if he understood some of the issues to do with AIDS patients, he would more readily come to terms with his own situation. Guy and the tutor agreed that he should leave the course and the tutor promised to talk to his manager about the reasons for this.

In the above example, Guy had every right to be upset. It was totally inappropriate for him to come on a course, with a very personal agenda, which was for professional discussion and learning. So often this is the case with the disruptive participant; they have some major problem that is exacerbated by sitting in a class discussing areas that are far too close to their own personal experience.

There are times when a participant appears to be disruptive for no particular reason. This happens more often in a course where the participant is bound to attend rather than choosing to attend. If an individual is not particularly interested in the subject, it can be a very pleasant game to be disruptive. In this situation the tutor has little choice but to confront the participant and ask them if they are prepared to work with the group or whether they would prefer to leave.

There is a belief that if the course is part of the overall training or education of a participant, then the tutor is bound to have that person in her class whether or not he or she is disruptive. This is simply not the case. The tutor can make it quite clear that there are ground rules for the group to work to and that if people do not wish to work to those ground rules, then they should not attend the sessions.

THE LATE ARRIVER

In many ways the late arriver is like the disruptive participant in that they appear to want attention. It may not be that they are angry, as the disruptive participant often is, but there is usually a very good reason why somebody is late over and over again. An example in one of the 'Help the Hospices' workshops was of a doctor on a course that included other doctors, nurses, social workers and a member of the clergy. This doctor arrived late at the start of the course and was late in arriving at several of the sessions, usually coming in with a lot of fuss. The first session was coloured by the individual arriving late and giving lengthy explanations as to what had happened on her way to the course.

The temptation is to play into the late arriver's hand by answering comments and getting involved, much to the annoyance to the rest of the group who arrived on time and would like to get on with the matter in hand. In many years of experience the only way to deal with the late arriver is to ignore them completely in terms of their arrival. This means that you do not recap on what has been happening in the few minutes that they have missed because this will feed what appears to be attention-seeking behaviour. Similarly, there should be no discussion about the time of arrival. Ideally, the tutor will continue with whatever was happening as if that person had not come into the room late and then, since the ploy is not working, the late participant will probably start coming on time.

The female doctor described who came late to several sessions and was completely ignored in terms of late arrival, though not in terms of contribution to the group, finally arrived at one session 15 minutes before it was due to start. The tutor was at the white board working out the next session from the original agenda and went on working at it though she nodded pleasantly to the individual. After a few seconds, the doctor said to the tutor, 'Can't you notice I'm early?' and the tutor smiled and said, 'I did notice, and I am pleased.' This doctor was never late again.

Whether an individual is a non-participator, an over-participator, disruptive or disruptive in being a late arriver, the outcome is usually a test of will between that individual and the tutor. If the tutor remains calm and continues to work with the group, very often the 'maverick' will begin to conform. It is important, however, always to explore why any member of a group behaves in an obviously different way from other group members. Sometimes it is simply that the individual needs to be different, but very often problems are identified and will need to be addressed.

THE HOSTILE GROUP

Perhaps the most difficult situation of all is when the group is hostile as a whole. Again, this seldom happens but when it does, it needs to be addressed sooner rather than later. It may be, for example, that the group is not pleased to be where it is. For example, members on a workshop away from their own clinical setting usually attend because that is what they want to do but occasionally a group might be set up by their manager who asks an outsider in to do some sessions with them. If the tutor finds such a group to be hostile, then there is little point in doing any work with that group until the hostility has been acknowledged and explored. This may take place as follows:

Tutor:	'I get the feeling that somehow as a group you are not happy because you are not participating well and certainly I don't feel that you are very pleased to see me. I wonder if we can look at this?' (Silence) 'Mary, would you like to tell me how you feel about being here?'
Mary:	'Well, I was sent. The manager came round and said she was getting this course put on for us and I'd got to come because I needed it.'
Sue:	'That's why I'm here. I was told I had to do it. I had to give up my days off to come here.'
John:	'Well, I felt I wasn't doing my job properly the way it was sold to me, two days with you on how to communicate. I don't think I've got any problems with communicating.'

The tutor found that each member of the group had been identified by a manager and sent on the course to improve their skills, almost as a punishment. The tutor had to negotiate with the group as follows:

Tutor:	'I'm sorry you feel the way you do and, yes, if you had to give up days off I can see that would irritate you, and certainly I can understand you being irritated if you've been made to feel that somehow you are not as effective as you could be. I am now faced with a difficult situation. We are in this lovely hotel, the weather is beautiful, I know from last night that the food is good – I wonder if we can make the best of the time we've got together and see what we can do that you will find useful?'

This approach worked with that group, primarily because it was then made clear that the only areas of communication that would be covered would be those that were identified by the participants with the exception of basic assessment. The group began to feel that they had some input into their two days and they felt, too, that they were being encouraged to use the time to their, rather than their manager's, advantage. This was of course an illusion because the areas that they wanted to explore were very much those that their manager had identified. What had gone wrong in this situation was that the manager had not recruited the staff in a sensitive way that would have left them feeling that they had some choice.

SUMMARY

In this chapter, a range of potential difficulties has been explored, which may occur in the teaching of communication skills. The tutor needs to be alert to identify such difficulties and to take swift but sensitive action.

CHAPTER EIGHT

Handling the cost of caring

Teaching health professionals to improve their ability to interact effectively with patients carries a cost for the participants in that when an individual interacts effectively and learns more about the other person, they
are very likely to get closer to that person's pain (Faulkner, 1992). Health
professionals are unlikely to disclose their reactions to patients' pain
because there is an implied belief that nurses and doctors need to be tough
in order to survive. This can cause conflict for the health professional who
wants to help their patients and their families to adapt to difficult
situations but who themselves want to feel comfortable. Often the conflict
is accompanied by guilt if there are feelings that could be labelled selfish.

In any course or workshop on effective interaction these issues need to
be addressed. A session on survival and support as part of the teacher's
agenda for the course/workshop will demonstrate that there is care for
the professionals as individuals. But it will also allow the individuals on
the course to discuss their own survival mechanisms. Covering this
material in a discussion session appears to be very effective, particularly
towards the end of the course/workshop, when the group members
have learned to trust each other and to share their thoughts and feelings.

PLANNING

In planning a session on support and survival, the aims need to be
identified and key questions formulated (Chapter 6). The aims may
include:

1. Helping individuals in the group to put a value on themselves;
2. Helping the individuals in the group to share their current coping
   mechanisms;
3. Encouraging discussion of the need for support at both a personal and
   a professional level.

Value on self

If student nurses are asked at the beginning of a course what they believe
to be the attributes of a 'good' nurse, they will list a number of attributes

most of which will be to do with giving (Tomlinson, 1985). This belief about what nursing is all about is reinforced in the clinical field and very often in the classroom. As a result a discussion session on survival and support will come as quite a surprise to many participants, be they nurses, doctors or other health professionals. In planning to meet the aims of putting a value on self, these beliefs of 'giving' must be taken into account for they could well put up barriers between what the health professional would like to disclose about their needs and what they are prepared to disclose.

Saying 'no' is often a problem for health professionals, particularly as they become more senior and feel that more is expected of them. In planning this session, care should be given to cover the area of setting limits on what any individual can do while still making time to be themselves.

Coping mechanisms

In planning this part of the discussion session questions need to be formulated to help people share the way that they cope at this time. This sharing will often lead to discussion and amusement as individuals think of different ways that they can relax when they are off-duty. Faulkner and Maguire (1988), in discussing the need for support, listed the following activities given by members of workshops:

1. Unwinding with a partner;
2. Going for long walks;
3. Alcohol;
4. Outside interests, for example, music, drama, hobbies;
5. Metaphorically kicking the cat;
6. Taking time out;
7. Talking to a supportive friend.

Most of these and more may come up in discussing coping mechanisms and the tutor needs to prepare to encourage disclosure of this type by appropriate questions.

Support

This part of the discussion session may need to be led by the tutor, with much more input than will be necessary for the first two components. This is because professional support is not very common and even when it is available there are often problems, as described by Booth and Faulkner (1986).

Personal support may well be raised as a coping mechanism when people are sharing their strategies for support. They may describe partners or friends to whom they can talk and share. This needs to be expected and, as a result, it will fall to the tutor to prepare input on guidelines for the setting up of professional support groups.

A key question in this part of the session will be to ask which members of the group have any form of professional support available to them. If a member of the group has such support then they should be encouraged to describe the mechanism, what works well about it and what could work better.

Finally, in planning the session, some examples for each area should be thought out by the tutor so that if there is any lack of response from the group there are examples that will start the discussion.

TIMING

If the session is going to adequately cover the areas of value on self, coping mechanisms and available support, then at least an hour should be allowed. An hour and a half gives much more time for discussion and leaves the group feeling that they have had a good opportunity to re-look at their own survival and coping mechanisms.

THE SESSION

The introduction of a discussion on survival and support is very important in order to set the ground rules for the session and also to encourage participants to realize that they too are important in the health care team. The introduction might proceed as follows:

Tutor: 'You'll all remember that at the beginning of this workshop I pointed out that I had some agenda items that I would not wish to leave the course without having covered. One of these was to do with you and what it costs you to look after people who are ill and frightened, and sometimes having difficulty accepting what is happening to them. What I'd like to do in this session is to ask you to share what works for you in that you can have hard and difficult days but still come back to work smiling the next day. And I want to cover this under three main headings. The first one is to do with you and your own worth, for too often in health care there is an implicit expectation that you will give and give and give. The Americans have a term for the result of that which is 'burn out'. So what we're doing today is looking at how we can avoid 'burn out'. That brings me to the second part of this session, which is to do with coping mechanisms that work for you. And we'll come back to that. But most of us have things that we can do to help us switch off. And, lastly, I want to look at the support network that you (a) have, and (b) feel that you don't have but would like. So, would someone like to start by talking about why they think we should put a value on us as well as on our patients?'

There may well be a pause after such an introduction while people look at each other, smile a bit and perhaps start the session off with a question. What the tutor needs to do is to remember that what she is aiming for is that participants will see that they do have a right to care for themselves. The following is an excerpt from a dialogue with a group of doctors and nurses:

Sandy: 'I think it's more important that other people put a value on us than we do on ourselves. You know, when I've been working all day and I'm ready to go home and then I'm asked if I can stay a bit longer, obviously I'm not very valued at all.'

Tutor: 'I'd like to come back to that, but I do want to start on a positive note and in the belief that we all have a responsibility to care for ourselves. So, would anyone else like to come in on this?'

Paul: 'I think Sandy's right. I value me but I can't always persuade other people to do it. But I'm getting better. Last week I was asked if I'd come in on my day off and I said, "I'm sorry, I can't do that." I felt very guilty afterwards.'

Tutor: 'I wonder if any of you have read the book *When I Say No, I Feel Guilty* [Smith, 1975]. I'll give you the reference later, but it's a good read. I wonder why we do feel *so* bad when we put our needs at the top of a list?'

Mary: 'Well, there's always someone there to show you up, isn't there? Someone who's always there before everybody else in the morning and still there when we all go home. That makes you feel bad.'

In this exchange students are highlighting their own reality in terms of how difficult it is to say 'no' and to put a value on their own needs. If the session starts off with these negative comments then the tutor needs to allow the feelings to be expressed and to pick up on any anger that is washing around so that it can be defused. It is then useful to go back to the negative statements and use them to look for a way forward.

Tutor: 'Sandy, you said earlier that you can't value yourself because nobody else does, and we've had one or two people supporting that. But we've also had one or two people giving us examples of when they do put a value on themselves. And this is often done by saying no. I wonder if you can think of a way forward when people devalue you?'

Sandy: 'I've been thinking about it, and I suppose we get what we ask for. I'm always prepared to stay on. So I guess it's as much me as them. But I really don't think I could say no.'

Tutor: 'It sounds as if you feel pretty indispensable.'

Sandy: 'Well, I guess I do. And yes, I know, I'm often in trouble at home because I'm home late and my wife says that she feels like a single parent. I guess I owe it to her to make more effort. I'd like to be sure that there won't be any re-criminations if I start being a little bit more selfish.'

Paul: 'You might find that your colleagues are appreciative. If you do work as long as you say then you're going to be making them all feel guilty if they do go home on time.' (Laughter)

The laughter resulting from Paul's comment was kindly and showed the level of sharing and comment possible in a group where there was mutual trust. Many participants leave such a session determined that they will get a better balance between what they give to their work and what they give to their family and loved ones.

Moving on to a sharing of coping mechanisms will usually lighten the atmosphere following the comments on valuing self. The tutor might start this section of the session by asking for people to share. For example:

Tutor: 'Well, I wonder if we can move on to looking at the things that help you to cope, and they may be many and various so I hope you will be feeling able to share. Who'd like to start?'

Ann: 'Do you mean like having a gin when you go home?' (Laughter)

Tutor: 'Yes, if that's what works for you. Let's put it down: alcohol. Anyone else?'

Dick: 'Well, I usually take my gin and have a bath and lock the door. And that gives me a good half-hour to wind down between work and home, because I live quite near to the hospice.'

Sally: 'But that's important too, isn't it? I live about two miles from the hospice and I often walk to work and back, and the walk from home to work lets me get my mind in gear but I'm always careful that when I walk home I just let the breezes blow and clear my mind. Then I can go home feeling a lot better.'

In this exchange participants were happy to share what worked for them. This part of the session is usually light-hearted but very useful in that it gives a wide range of activities that are seen to be therapeutic in terms of making the break between work and home.

The section of the session that is concerned with support does carry small risks in that if there are people within the group who feel that they do not have support they may be very bitter. In addition, where this is also true of people feeling that they are not valued, the support section must be followed by a lighter note before the session is complete. Individuals may give glowing accounts of personal support that could make other people feel rather upset.

Faulkner (1992) gives the example of driving home from work, feeling that when she got there, there would be a husband who would open the car door, pour her a gin and tonic and hear about her day. But when she got home he opened the car door and said, 'Thank goodness you're home! wait till you know what a *day* I have had!' This example demonstrates that even if there is a supportive partner they do not always meet their loved one's needs. Such an illustration is not meant to degrade personal support mechanisms but rather to show that support is a two-way exchange and that sometimes there will be competing needs between partners, friends or any couple who help each other with difficulties in their personal lives.

Similarly with professional support, members of the group will give very varying examples of what, if any, professional support is available to them. The aim of this session may be to identify both formal and informal professional support mechanisms. But it may not be that anyone in the group can offer examples of either. Booth and Faulkner (1986) describe the difficulties of attempting to set up support groups and showed that no matter the grade of health professional, there are difficulties in admitting to the need for support.

What can be done in such a situation is to set out the ground rules for a support group that will be effective and to hope that members of the group will go back to their own clinical setting and think about setting up a group that will be useful. Faulkner and Maguire (1988) set out a number of ground rules, as follows:

1. Confidentiality within the group must be assured. It requires only one group member to gossip outside and trust is lost as each member wonders who broke faith.
2. Problems raised must be professional and relate to work. This avoids embarrassment to those who might disclose highly personal matters in the group but regret it later.
3. Linked to point 2, the group must not be used for catharsis.
4. The group is not to be used for personal therapy unless this is agreed to be its function by all members and the group is led by a trained psychotherapist.
5. The leader must be experienced in group methods and dynamics and be capable of ensuring that discussions are not too superficial or too damaging.

6. The leader ensures that no one member monopolizes the group, including him/herself.

Even if no-one in the group has access to a professional support group, setting out the above ground rules will usually engender considerable discussion and questioning about where, for example, one finds a leader, and how many people should be in the group. And although in a workshop this cannot be taken further in terms of starting a support group, ideas will have been planted which may come to fruition and be described at follow-up days.

CONCLUDING THE SESSION

The session needs to be brought to a close in a very positive way by making a checklist on the board. For example, a list of all the helpful elements in terms of survival. It is important to acknowledge and to thank the group for sharing their own particular mechanisms for support. If there have been members of the group who have shown that they have difficulties in gaining support, then this needs to be acknowledged and perhaps an open question asked of the group as follows:

Tutor: 'I've had the sense through this session that some of you are pretty short on day-to-day support. I wonder if anyone would like to make comment on whether this session has been of use to them?'

Such a question gives the members of the group the chance to give feedback on what they have found useful and also to verbalize what they might do when they go back to their own clinical field. This is one of those situations where the tutor does not always know how useful such a session has been. But it is not unusual following workshops of this type to have a letter which perhaps says how valuable it was to think of ways forward and to let the tutor know that a support group has started, or that an individual is finding it easier to say 'no'. This sort of feedback can be very rewarding.

POTENTIAL PROBLEMS

It is possible, although very rare, that members of a group in discussing the cost of caring may demonstrate that one of them may be having difficulties in coping. This may show in terms of a group member being very quiet throughout the session, or showing signs of distress. In either of these situations the tutor should pick up on the problem to check out whether indeed the silence or distress or other manifestation is linked in any way with the discussion. The following exchange illustrates one example of such a problem.

Tutor: 'Well, most of you have given very interesting and very useful ways of surviving, from Dick's gin in a long, hot bath – in a locked bathroom I note – through to Sally's walk in the fresh air, blowing away the cobwebs, and all sorts of things in between. Doreen, I notice that you haven't actually said what works for you.'

Doreen: 'I'm not sure that anything does.'

Tutor: 'That sounds fairly serious. Do you want to talk about that here?'

Doreen: 'I don't want to talk about it anywhere.'

After this Doreen got up and left the room, and the tutor asked if someone would go with her to check that she was all right. Later, on a one-to-one basis, Doreen admitted to the tutor that although she had come in to this area of care she felt very much alone. Her marriage had broken up, her children were grown up and moved away, and so she threw herself into her work and became unpopular because she was over-working. She was always there first thing in the morning, and always the last to go home at night.

In this instance the tutor gave advice on talking this through with someone in her own clinical area to see if there was a way forward. The problem here is that the tutor may be tempted to get into therapeutic mode, even though this is seldom useful, in an attempt to help. However, since the problem is in the individual's own clinical area it needs to be resolved with the people concerned, and perhaps with the help of a general practitioner if the problem is such that the individual needs to have some 'time out'.

It could be argued that Doreen's problem might surface in any teaching session. Such problems are discussed in Chapter 7. The point here is that in a group where most people appear to have very good mechanisms for making the distinction between work and play, then the person who is not coping can feel more desolate than usual and have feelings of failure in terms of 'If they're all coping, why can't I?'

The other problem that is likely to surface in such a session is the personal issue problem. Again, this can surface in any teaching session but in terms of coping and surviving in a demanding job, personal issues may be raised as a reason for needing more support than others. This, again, is discussed in Chapter 7.

SUMMARY

In this chapter, the responsibility has been seen for accepting that when individuals improve their communication skills they will get closer to their patient's pain, and that this does have cost. A discussion session has been outlined to pick up both the costs of caring and to examine some of the ways that members of the group cope by:

1. putting a value on self;
2 describing coping mechanisms that allow them to make a break between work and play;
3. discussing support at both a personal and professional level.

It has been seen that such a session might elicit problems for members of the group who feel that they are not coping very well with the cost of caring, or who feel that personal issues are getting in the way.

REFERENCES

Booth, K. and Faulkner, A. (1986) Problems encountered in setting up support groups in nursing. *Nurse Education Today*, **6**, 244–51.
Faulkner, A. (1992) *Effective Interaction with Patients*, Churchill Livingstone, Edinburgh.
Faulkner, A. and Maguire, P. (1988) The need for support. *Nursing*, **5** (28), 1010–12.
Smith, M. (1975) *When I Say No, I Feel Guilty*, Dial Press, New York.
Tomlinson, A. (1985) *CINE Report No. 3 (South)*, Health Education Authority report, London.

CHAPTER NINE

Evaluation

The traditional way to measure the effects of learning is to examine the participants of the course, giving a pass or fail result with credits and distinctions for those who do really well. Such a system inevitably puts participants in competition with each other in terms of a hierarchy of progress. What an examination seldom does is to give the participant any feedback on those areas in which they have done very well and those areas in which they need to improve before their marks get better.

Evaluation can take a much wider view of the effects of teaching and, depending on the method of evaluation used, can be of benefit to both the participant and to the tutor. The type of evaluation will depend on the aims of the study sessions, the group and the time available.

INFORMAL EVALUATION

Informal evaluation is often used at the end of a study day or a short workshop, where the aim may be more to do with the raising of awareness of the need to improve standards than it is to actually improve skills. There is a double benefit to the participant in that (1) they can consider what they have actually gained from their study, and (2) they are encouraged to give an opinion on the quality and appropriateness of the material that they have received. For the tutors to the course, informal evaluation gives feedback on the material covered and the methods used. Evaluation comments can then be used to improve future study days, courses or workshops. Informal evaluation may be either open, where members of a group are encouraged to talk about the course and what they have gained from it, or written, where the course participants are invited to write down their reactions to the course.

Open evaluation

As with any interactive session, open evaluation will work best with a group of less than 20 participants who, preferably, have been learning together for long enough for there to be knowledge and trust within the group. A structure that works reasonably well is to ask a number of questions to which course participants will respond. These questions should follow the positive model that has been shown throughout this book, that is, questions about positive aspects of the work should be asked before negative ones. Figure 9.1 shows questions which will allow participants to comment on all aspects of the course. The tutor will note down all comments for future reference.

---

1. What aspects of the course have you found most useful?

2. What aspects of the course have you found least useful?

3. What suggestions have you for improving the course?

4. How satisfactory were the domestic arrangements?

5. How satisfactory was the teaching environment?

6. What comments would you like to make about the teaching team?

7. Have you any other comments to make about the course?

Figure 9.1   Questions for informal open evaluation.

The alternative to defined questions is an open approach which says to the participants, 'Please make any comments that you feel are appropriate.' The difficulty with that approach is that participants will almost always list only those areas where they have been unhappy about what has happened. By encouraging a positive response the participants will be encouraged to think of gains from the teaching while knowing that they are also going to have an opportunity to talk about potential improvements.

In many ways one could argue that if the teaching has been well directed and the students a trusting group, many if not all potential problems will have been picked up during the course of the work. Even if this is the case, the end of the course evaluation acts as a useful summary for people to take away with them. One very strong argument against open informal evaluation is that individuals will not feel able to be honest about areas where they were not happy. This does not seem to be the case in a considerable experience of working for two to three days with a group and then asking for their opinion, although the tutor may have to encourage disclosure of problems. The following type of exchange is not unusual:

Tutor:	'Well, thank you all, you've been very positive about the useful aspects of the course. I wonder now if you'd like to tell me those parts of the course that you haven't found quite so useful?'
Jenny:	'I think I found it all useful.'
Tutor:	'That's very gratifying. Does anyone feel less positive? I have broad shoulders and know that none of us get it right all the time.'
Joe:	'Well, I did wonder why you left us in our small groups to talk about spiritual issues. It seemed as though you weren't giving it quite the importance that you gave to other areas.'
Mary:	'I felt that. In fact I felt that even on the agenda spiritual issues wasn't very important.'
Tutor:	'I'm sorry you felt like that. Can somebody suggest how this could be handled differently in future?'
Joe:	'I can. After all, with many of our discussion sessions you obviously had clear questions for us to consider. And that helped. It gave us a structure for the discussion. But with the spiritual issues you just asked us to discuss problems that we'd had and then feed back to you what had happened. It all seemed a little flat.'
Tutor:	'Thank you for being so honest, Joe. I'll take that on board for future workshops.'

In the above exchange there had to be some encouragement to make the negative comments and to move on to helpful suggestions. Occasionally the reverse is true, when a situation arises in which a member of the group who has not found the course or workshop to be as they expected. They may try to interrupt positive comments with negative ones. Again, this seldom happens because such dissatisfaction should have been picked up earlier. If there are negative elements, then, before the group leaves, the tutor should try and talk to the individual/s and find out why they have waited until the end of the workshop to share their dissatisfaction.

Written evaluation

There are a number of points to consider about written evaluation. Not least *when* it should be completed. Ideally it should be completed at the end of the course/workshop or study day and the forms collected before participants leave. There is, however, an alternative argument that participants should be given time to think over the value of the day, or the course or workshop, and then fill in the form and return it to the course organizer. The difficulty with this latter view is that the response rate is usually reasonably low. Another issue about written evaluation is whether or not participants should be asked to sign their names. The view here is that if the evaluation remains anonymous individuals will feel much more free to be totally honest about their feelings.

The questions asked on a written evaluation need be no different from those asked at an open evaluation, although there is more room to manoeuvre. For example, the written evaluation can be a 'tick list' of questions where participants give a score, as in Figure 9.2. The advantage to this is that the material from a whole group can be more readily collated, but there is the disadvantage that there is no opportunity for the student to make specific comments about areas of concern to them. Even

Communication in Health Care

Evaluation of Study Day

Please tick the appropriate column for each question and return to course tutor. Thank you.

Teaching sessions	Very useful	Useful	Not sure	Not useful	Totally useless
1. Keynote address Communication issues in health care					
2. Video demonstration					
3. Small group work					
4. Session 1 Towards a team approach					
5. Session 2 Communication: The future					
Organizational aspects	Very good	Good	Not sure	Poor	Very poor
1. Teaching environment					
2. Standard of teaching					
3. Domestic arrangements					
4. Catering arrangements					

Figure 9.2 'Tick list' type of evaluation form.

if a space is left at the bottom for general comments, it does not tend to bring out quite the wealth of information that open questions do.

In terms of signing or leaving the evaluation form blank, it is possible to give participants a choice and also to explain to them the value of owning comments. This requires the tutor to negotiate with the group. Perhaps as follows:

Tutor: 'Before we finish the course, I'd like to talk to you about evaluation forms which I'm going to ask you to complete. Many of you have already commented to me about how you feel about this particular workshop and may feel that evaluation now is not really necessary. However, what I'm going to put to you is that if you will fill the form in for me, it will help us both. It gives you a chance to concentrate your thoughts on what was most useful to you, and what would have been even more useful in constructive comment. It also helps me, because although every group is different, often the things that are not appropriate for one group are equally inappropriate for another. It may be, for example, that the way a particular subject is approached didn't grab you in the way it might have if it had been handled differently. That's the sort of thing I need to know from you. There is a space at the bottom of the form for your name, but you do have the freedom not to fill it in. The only thing I would say about that is that if you feel that the comments you're making are useful I'd appreciate it if you could own those comments. There's going to be no retribution to anyone who hasn't enjoyed particular aspects of this workshop, but I certainly will be helped by your honesty. So can you, at this break, pick up an evaluation form and that gives you lunchtime to fill it in. And I'd like to collect them sometime after lunch, before you all go away. Thank you.'

Such negotiation often brings comments from the group and sometimes it brings a request to also have the chance for verbal feedback. Certainly both verbal and written feedback can be used together if the group members feel that there are things they need to say as a participant, for example.

FORMAL EVALUATION

Informal evaluation gives the group and the tutor a chance to talk about issues to do with satisfaction about the course and also to look with insight into what they feel they have gained. What it does not do is give participants any indication of how or if their skills have improved. In measuring the skills of communication, written work is unlikely to give any measure of an individual's ability to interact effectively with a patient. Methods of measuring skills have generally come from research initiatives, and the difficulty here is that the measures are often far too complex to be used for a group of participants at the end of a workshop or course. It can be seen in Chapter 5 that audio feedback can be a powerful teaching tool. It can also be seen in Chapter 10 that rating audio-tapes has been a very effective method of measuring skills.

In fact it is possible to evaluate learning by giving students some global feedback on their progress from an audio-tape made at the beginning of a course and that made at the end. A decision has to be made first as to what type of feedback the participant requires. If, for example, the feedback is on skills then a tutor can listen to part of a tape and pick out those skills that are being used effectively. A short written global report could then be given to each participant showing their skills had improved from the beginning of the course to the end. The problem here is that such an exercise can be very time-consuming. One has to consider alternatives.

One alternative to the tutor listening to parts of a tape (Chapter 5) is to ask the participants themselves to transcribe both the tape they make at the beginning of a course or workshop and the tape they make at the end. They are then asked to pick out from that transcript areas where they feel they have improved from the beginning to the end. The tutor needs to give guidelines for the student to use (Figure 9.3), and then mark the resulting evaluation, by checking the participants' comments against the transcript and either endorsing or correcting the comments made. This exercise can be very useful to participants because it will consolidate what they have learnt. If the skills have not been mastered, then the participant will be unable herself to pick out the good areas of practice, but can usually spot errors. The tutor can then give appropriate, positive feedback plus constructive advice for improvement.

The ideal situation in evaluating skills is that the student can see real differences in their performance. In the research study undertaken by Maguire and Faulkner (Faulkner, 1992) participants showed an improvement in definite areas such as an increased use of open questions and a decreased use of inappropriate reassurance. Even though there are other areas where improvement was not so noticeable, feedback of this type can be very beneficial to the participants. Another important element in this type of evaluation is that the participant is not in competition with other members of the group but only in competition with their own performance.

Experience has shown that participants become quite excited when they find that they are using skills more appropriately than when they started the course or the workshop. Their interest in other participants rotates around positive feedback so that other members also feel that

1. Make positive comment first on:

   (a) the extent to which you feel you have made a reasonable assessment of the patient

   (b) skills that you have used effectively

          e.g.   open questions
                       cue based
                       clarification
                       encouraging precision
                       educated guesses
                       opening gambits
                       losing gambits
                       facilitation

   (c) level of interaction you feel you have achieved

   (d) how clear and relevant your explanations were

2. Make constructive suggestions on how you hope to improve:

   (a) on overall assessment

   (b) on use of skills and addition of skills not evident

   (c) on reaching deeper level (if appropriate) and subsequent 'lifting'

   (d) on improving length, time and effectiveness of information giving

Figure 9.3 Guidelines for written feedback *from* students on transcripts of assessment interviews.

their own skills are improving. This can have a very motivating boost for the whole group who will wish to improve. The feedback they have given to each other during sessions on role play, audio feedback and, indeed, discussion topics underlines their confidence in their ability to improve skills and practice.

The best possible evaluation is that which includes both the informal and the formal elements. Unfortunately in many learning situations there is not time for both. Similarly, in some situations there is a demand for an examination situation. It is argued here that feedback on audio-tapes can take the place of the formal examination question when measuring a person's learning over the period of the course.

In a more formal setting such as a module as part of either nurse or medical education it may not always be possible for participants themselves to produce audio-tapes either at the beginning or the end of the course. What can show skills in a participant in this situation is to ask them to rate a transcript of an interaction. In this instance each participant would be given a transcript of an interaction between a health professional and a patient. In this they would be picking up those elements of the interaction that were effective and those that needed to be improved. Figure 9.4 shows guidelines for giving feedback on a transcribed interaction not made by the participant. What is important about the transcription is that it shows both effective and ineffective interaction, so encouraging the participants to think positively about that which needs improving. Such exercises can be given to participants to rate in their own time or it can be a class activity where each individual works on the transcript over a given period of time.

---

1. Give positive comments first on:

   (a) the extent to which a reasonable assessment has been made

   (b) skills used effectively

              e.g.   open questions
                           cue-based clarification
                           encouraging precision
                           educated guesses
                           opening gamb its
                           closing gambits
                           facilitation

   (c) level of interaction

   (d) clear, relevant explanations

2. Make constructive suggestions for improvement:

   (a) on overall assessment

   (b) on use of skills and addition of skills not evident

   (c) on reaching deeper level (if appropriate) and subsequent 'lifting'

   (d) on improving length, time and effectiveness of information giving

Figure 9.4 Guidelines for written feedback *to* students on transcripts of assessment interviews.

MEASURING EFFECTS OVER TIME

In teaching interactive skills and measuring whether they have improved during a workshop a question remains as to whether those skills will be integrated into the clinical arena and maintained over time. Ideally, in training for nurses, doctors and other health professionals, interactive skills would be part of the curriculum in every module. In this way each module could top-up skills in the context of the specialty of the module. This would encourage generalization of skills. In workshops held for trained health professionals there is not always that capacity for continual top-up. The most effective workshops are those that have a follow-up day or two days six months or so after the original. This allows people to come back and talk about what has worked for them and to identify areas where they still need help. Also, if audio-tapes are used as a gauge of skill, it can be an opportunity for the participant to make another tape-recorded interaction and again have some global feedback on whether their skills have been maintained, improved or in fact have deteriorated over time.

Another possibility is that at the end of a course or workshop participants should be given the opportunity for distance-learning. This will require a contract between participants and the tutors to determine what sort of distance-learning takes place.

It may be, for example, that participants contract to send in tape recordings of interactions with patients at clearly defined intervals. The tutor will then contract to send global feedback of progress. The other alternative is that the students contract to rate transcripts which the tutor will send them. And again there will be clearly defined times for receiving transcripts and for sending them back and for gaining feedback. In research terms the effects of distance-learning, in interactive skills, have still to be evaluated. In day-release courses at Trent Palliative Care Centre there has been a variety of responses from those participants who are prepared to send in tapes for global feedback and those that have felt unable to do so. At present the numbers taking advantage of this option are small but it is hoped that the effect of distance-learning on maintaining skills over time will be measured at a later date.

SUMMARY

In this chapter evaluation has been considered as a method of giving both student and tutors feedback and reinforcement on the value of teaching interactive skills. It has been argued that open or written feedback can give some indication of satisfaction with learning material and also positive suggestions for improvement of future courses. This, however, does not show increments of learning in participants.

Formal measurement of skills has been considered following research to measure skills by rating audio-taped interviews. Suggestions as to how the scientific measures can be adapted to give global feedback to participants have been given, along with the notion that it requires that a participant can recognize the skills in order to rate them. It has been suggested that participants can have a measure of their progress through rating transcripts of interactions that they have themselves not been involved in. Finally, the problem of maintaining skills over time has been covered briefly, with the suggestion that distance-learning (Chapter 1) may be the way forward for the future.

REFERENCE

Faulkner, A. (1992) The evaluation of training programmes for communication skills in palliative care. *Journal of Cancer Care*, **1**(2), 75–9.

PART THREE

Learning from Research

CHAPTER TEN

The need to teach effective interaction strategies

It is well documented by many authors (for example, Ashworth, 1980; Faulkner, 1980; Macleod Clark, 1982; Maguire, Roe, Goldberg et al., 1978) that health professionals do not possess the skills necessary for interacting effectively with patients and their families. In this respect the volume of research identified a problem that could not be ignored, because of the number of studies with similar results.

In 1980 the Health Education Council (HEC) funded the Communication in Nurse Education project (CINE), which resulted from the enthusiasm of Jane Randell (HEC), Jill Macleod Clark (King's College, London) and Ann Faulkner (University of Manchester). The aims of the study were to develop means of teaching basic communication skills to nurse learners in the first 18 months of their basic general training and to evaluate the programme by using a pre-test/post-test design and control groups (Faulkner and Macleod Clark, 1987).

There were also two national surveys; one of directors of nurse education and one of nurse tutors. The aim of the first survey was to identify, in each school, (1) the commitment to teaching specific communication courses, (2) the place of teaching communication skills within basic training and (3) the attitudes held by directors of nurse education towards communication. There was an 84% response to this survey, which suggested that the results would give a representative view on how directors of nurse education perceived communication as part of the curriculum. The directors of nurse education survey was also used to identify schools of nursing willing to take part in the CINE project (Faulkner, 1986). The second survey was a modified version of the first, sent to those tutors who were responsible for teaching communication skills. There was a 75% response rate to this questionnaire.

THE SURVEYS

The surveys were designed to elicit information about the teaching of communication skills in schools and colleges of nursing, midwifery and health visiting. Questions were asked about the importance of teaching communication as a separate subject, about the commitment in terms of time and expertise given to the subject, the amount of aids and audio-visual equipment available to tutors, and (of particular importance) the preparation of tutors required to give them the skills to teach effective communication to their students.

The findings from both groups had a very high level of agreement. However, the responses to the tutors' questionnaire gave a much more realistic picture of the difficulties encountered in putting communication as a subject into the curriculum. It was interesting that in Scotland, 65% of tutors were engaged in teaching communication skills but only 36% felt that they had had adequate preparation to take on such teaching. In the rest of Britain, 97% of tutors were actively engaged in teaching communication skills but only 73% had had some training in teaching the subject. Overall, less than 5% of tutors felt that they were totally prepared to teach communication skills to their students. Directors of nurse education, on the other hand, felt that probably only 2% of their staff had had any preparation for teaching communication skills.

There were many contradictions in the responses to the main body of the questionnaire. For example, 95% of respondents felt that communication was an important subject that should be taught, yet little time appeared to be allocated to such teaching. Many felt that 5% of curriculum time was a realistic figure, although some respondents put this at 10%. Even at this level it can be seen that communication, in reality, had a low priority compared to the medical specialties that are taught to nurses throughout their training.

The findings from the survey reinforced the CINE team's belief that the project was worthwhile and necessary. The full results can be seen in the CINE report of the survey (Faulkner, 1986).

THE CINE TEACHING PROGRAMME

Over the length of the entire CINE project four tutors were recruited. These were Christine Fessey, Brian Neeson, Anne Tomlinson and Anne Williams. They were trained to teach communication skills by the project directors, Ann Faulkner and Jill Macleod Clark, and with a commitment from Will Bridge and Jane Randell. The programme for teaching was based on a micro skills approach (see Chapter 11). However, the tutors soon found that teaching the skills was a small part of their work compared with 'selling' the idea of the CINE project to the schools of nursing which volunteered to take part. Negotiating time and space and the ability to teach students in small groups was a time-consuming exercise and also a learning exercise in terms of asserting beliefs in the project.

The findings of this study (Faulkner and Macleod Clark, 1987) showed improvements in students' perceptions, attitudes, skills and knowledge in relation to communication in both the control and experimental groups. It was gratifying to find that the students in the experimental groups demonstrated substantially greater increments in learning than did the students in the control group. One area in which this was particularly noticeable was in the area of understanding and gaining knowledge of the complexity of communication, and to the reactions and skills displayed when faced with threatening or emotionally loaded situations. Paradoxically, the students in the experimental groups felt less confident of their ability to communicate well at the end of their teaching experience than did the control groups. It could be argued that in learning more about the complexity of effective communication, the students were much harder on themselves in terms of what they expected.

PHASE II – PREPARATION FOR TEACHERS

Given the results of the surveys and the findings from the CINE teaching, a second phase of the project was funded with the aim of exploring the problems of helping nurse tutors acquire the knowledge and skills to teach communication effectively. Access was gained to two institutions with a tutor training programme, with a view to negotiating part of the curriculum to update tutor students' communication skills and to develop experiential teaching methods.

Not surprisingly, the tutor students' communication skills needed considerable updating before they could be taught to use experimental methods. The programme was well accepted and in at least one of the two programmes the communication element was incorporated into the curriculum for future courses.

There are many parallels between the findings of the CINE project and other work undertaken in the field. Faulkner and Maguire (1984) found that audio feedback training of nurses caring for mastectomy patients had a beneficial effect on the skills of many of the nurses in the study. These skills were generally inadequate before teaching took place but improved more in ward staff where there was group cohesion and support than they did in the community, where many nurses felt that they were working in isolated situations.

A further study funded by the Cancer Research Campaign (CRC) aimed to teach community nurses in groups to improve their interactive skills (Maguire, Faulkner and Fairbairn, 1989). In this study similar results were found to those of the ward staff in Faulkner and Maguire's study, though the level of improvement was not entirely satisfactory overall.

WORKSHOPS

In addition to research which aimed to put in a teaching intervention, other initiatives were undertaken in an attempt to improve interactive skills in health professionals. The Royal College of Nursing negotiated to put on workshops for nurses involved in cancer care. These were originally mounted by Gaynor Nurse and Ann Faulkner (unpublished) and lasted three days. The Extramural Department at the University of Manchester administered the first course, which was subsequently repeated annually by popular request.

A major problem with these first workshops was the fact that they were for nurses only because, repeatedly, the participants would alibi poor practice by blaming doctors for their problems. Peter Maguire (Manchester) was involved in the teaching of these courses and shared the concern of teaching nurses alone. When Gaynor Nurse retired, Faulkner and Maguire took over the courses and moved towards making them multidisciplinary. They also refined and developed their teaching methods and worked towards a common model of patient assessment and of strategies to help health professionals deal adequately with patients' needs for psychosocial care.

Another initiative in the early 1980s came from Help the Hospices, a small charity committed to improving palliative care in the hospice world. These workshops (Maguire and Faulkner, 1988) followed a similar pattern to the Extramural Department courses but were five rather than three days long. Repeatedly, at informal evaluation, participants requested that they should come back at a later date to review progress. As a result, both the Extramural Department and Help the Hospices workshops are followed by a two-day follow-up six months after the first part has been completed.

One of the difficulties of teaching communication skills on short workshops is the lack of feedback to tutors on what has been achieved. Feedback from participants on both the Extramural Department and Help the Hospices workshops was enthusiastic and positive, but it did not show if skills had been (1) improved or (2) maintained over time. Further, they did not validate teaching methods except in terms of comfort and satisfaction with the way the course was taught.

The need to move from informal evaluation to a more scientific mode of measuring the effects of the courses became a priority. After much discussion, Maguire and Faulkner developed a protocol which was subsequently funded as part of the Cancer Research Campaign Psychological Medicine Group's programme (Faulkner, 1992).

The aim of the new project was to evaluate the effects of short workshops on communication skills and to validate the teaching methods used. As with the CINE project, a pre/post post-test design was used, with participants being asked to interview a simulated patient at the beginning of a workshop, at the end of a workshop, and again six months later at follow-up. The evidence to date shows that teaching methods have been validated and that there is improvement in the skills of participants from the beginning to the end of each workshop.

THE CASCADE PROJECT

An interesting and unexpected aspect to the Help the Hospice workshops was the interest shown by many participants in themselves mounting courses on teaching communication skills. These individuals appeared to particularly appreciate the fact that the courses were taught by a nurse/doctor team, and wanted to emulate this multidisciplinary approach.

As a result of this interest, in teaching in their own locality, Help the Hospices funded a project aimed to generate a cascade effect from the Faulkner/Maguire model. Pairs of teachers were given an intensive workshop on developing skills in teaching communication and were then supported in their efforts to put on courses and to improve their teaching skills. The tutors in the project came back for follow-up six months after their initial course and reported progress and problems that they had encountered.

An initial difficulty encountered in the Cascade Project was the level of knowledge, attitudes and skills of the participants. They were by definition a self-selected group but in the early days it was found that if the participants had not attended a basic skills course this could lead to problems in dealing with the teaching material because they themselves were not comfortable with their own skills. This again parallels the findings with the tutor students in the CINE Phase II project and perhaps encompasses the problems of many health professionals who, having been through both their basic and post-basic training, have never had formal teaching on the skills of effective communication. As a result of these problems, it had to be made a condition of attendance that participants had either attended a Faulkner/Maguire course or had a similar background learning experience before they attended the teaching workshop.

Less intensive teaching courses for individuals who wish to improve their ability to teach are regularly supported by Help the Hospices. Many of those attending have also requested and successfully found a place on the Cascade teaching courses with a professional partner. These partnerships are not always doctor–nurse, but can be doctor–nurse, doctor–social worker, nurse–social worker or any combination of health professionals. The notion of the doctor–nurse, or similar, team is that there is a wider perspective brought to the teaching, given that the backgrounds of the two tutors complement and enhance each other.

The Cascade Project was completed in 1991, by which time there were approximately 20 pairs of teachers around the country committed to setting up their own courses, some with more success than others. There was, however, an expressed need for those teachers to continue to be supported in their efforts to build on their expertise. Help the Hospices has funded a support programme for these teachers which gives them access to someone who will help if requested, and also gives them a chance to meet other tutors and share their problems and their successes. A north and south support group have been set up and the effect of this is being evaluated.

LEARNING FROM RESEARCH

It has been noted that there are many parallels between the CINE project and other initiatives. This includes the CRC-funded evaluation and validation study (Faulkner, 1992). There are, however, some significant differences. Perhaps the greatest difference is the approach to teaching. In the CINE project a micro skills approach was used and found to be quite appropriate to student nurses as part of their basic curriculum. However, as the sessions moved on, a more strategy-based approach was used to consolidate the learning of the skills.

In the workshops that have been evaluated in the CRC project, a much more general view is taken of communication and the skills are teased out of the general strategy being taught. For example, when teaching assessment skills, which is a major part of these workshops, the appropriate skills are all identified in the same session. What is common here is that both projects showed that if there is a commitment to teaching effective interaction in health care then there will be positive outcomes from that. Several similarities arise.

1. The teaching methods for both the CINE project and for the Extra-mural Department/Help the Hospice workshops are very similar in that they depend heavily on interactive teaching processes. In Part One of this book the examples given are related primarily to the Maguire/Faulkner (1988) approach, but each method can also be used to teach micro skills.
2. In both projects the skills of the learners have been found, generally, to be inadequate at the beginning of the course and to have improved at the end. The important point here is that this includes many of those who are being expected to teach communication skills. A lesson learned has been that before anyone is taught how to develop their ability to teach communication skills, they must have a top-up on their own ability to interact effectively with patients and their families.

3. In both the CINE and the CRC project it was found that people who teach the skills of communication do need support in their work. This is because interactive teaching is much more demanding and draining than straight lecturing.
4. Both the projects have shown that measurement of skills is possible, both at a macro and micro level. Current work at the Trent Palliative Care Centre is aimed at making the scale developed for the CRC project (Faulkner, 1992) a much more manageable tool for measuring at tutor to student level.

SUMMARY

In this chapter the problems of communication between health professionals and their patients have been considered at several levels. First, research has been described to show that health professionals, in general, do not have the necessary interactive skills to help their patients. Second, projects have been described that moved on from identifying the problem to intervention studies with the hope of developing methods of teaching that will be generalizable to other areas.

Particular emphasis has been given to the CINE project and the CRC evaluation project. Initiatives have been described that show the growing commitment of both funding bodies and health professionals to the improvement of communication skills, and it has been rewarding to have senior doctors, nurses and social workers recognize that they need to attend courses aimed to improve their skills.

Overall it has been demonstrated that: (1) research findings have highlighted the need for effective teaching of communication skills; (2) that methods described in this book have been validated; and (3) that measurement of skills is possible. There is much work still to be done, particularly in perfecting a measurement tool that can be used by tutors for evaluation in basic training courses.

REFERENCES

Ashworth, P. (1980) *Care to Communicate*, Royal College of Nursing, London.
Faulkner, A. (1980) The student nurse's role in giving information to patients. Unpublished M. Litt thesis. University of Aberdeen.
Faulkner, A. (1986) *A Survey of Schools of Nursing*, Report to Health Education Council, London.
Faulkner, A. (1992) The evaluation of training programmes for communication skills in palliative care. *Journal of Cancer Care*, 1(2), 75–8.
Faulkner, A. and Macleod Clark, J. (1987) Communication skills teaching in nurse education, in *Nursing Education: Research and Development* (ed. B. Davis), Croom Helm, London.

Faulkner, A. and Maguire, P. (1984) Teaching assessment skills, in *Recent Advances in Nursing: Communication* (ed. A. Faulkner), Churchill Livingstone, Edinburgh.

Maguire, P. and Faulkner, A. (1988) How to improve the counselling skills of doctors and nurses in cancer care. *British Medical Journal*, **297**, 847–9.

Maguire, P., Faulkner, A. and Fairbairn, S. (1989) *Training Community Nurses to Assess and Monitor Patients with Cancer*, Report to the Cancer Research Campaign, London.

Macleod Clark, J. (1982) Nurse–patient verbal interaction. Unpublished PhD thesis. University of London.

Maguire, P., Roe, P., Goldberg, D. *et al.* (1978) The value of feedback in teaching interviewing skills to medical students. *Psychological Medicine*, **8**, 695–704.

CHAPTER ELEVEN

The skills of communication

Given that there is agreement that the skills of communication need to be taught to health professionals, then a decision has to be made as to how those skills are going to be taught. In the CINE programme (Faulkner and Macleod Clark, 1987) the emphasis was on teaching micro skills and then linking those skills to nursing practice. The Maguire/Faulkner model (Maguire and Faulkner, 1988) depends more on teaching strategies to help the health professional to interact effectively with their patients, and skills are teased out throughout the workshops.

These two methods of teaching skills are not mutually exclusive. For example, student nurses, who will have to learn that there are considerable differences between social and professional interaction, can benefit enormously from a grounding in micro skills which then moves on to strategies that incorporate those skills. The Maguire/Faulkner (1988) model can then build on the skills that individuals bring to a workshop, but can also use expertise within the group for maximum learning and development.

TEACHING MICRO SKILLS

In the CINE project 15 sessions were negotiated for teaching micro skills during the first 18 months of training. Two of the sessions were used to introduce communication to students. Six sessions were spent on skills of communication, and seven sessions were spent on combining skills with nursing practice. Figure 11.1 shows the content of the 15 sessions.

Each of the CINE sessions was negotiated for two hours and each of those two-hour sessions contained a 15-minute tea break. Some sessions, however, had to be contained within one hour, which did have an effect on the type of teaching involved. Teaching methods included lecture, exercises, discussion, role play and use of video material and vignettes of different situations.

One of the difficulties of teaching micro skills in this way is that it takes several sessions before the teaching is linked directly to nursing practice. This is important since one of the first things that student nurses and medical students, for example, need to grasp is the fundamental

Session 1
The place, importance and relevance of communication in nursing
An introduction to communication, human needs, health education and the skills required for effective communication including understanding self and others, attitudes, culture variables etc

Session 2
Elements of communication
Detailed breakdown of the verbal and non-verbal components of communication and skills needed for effective communication

Session 3
Questioning
Obtaining information, assessing patients, types of questioning, purpose of each type, knowing appropriate use of each

Session 4
Listening and attending
Listening habits, hearing, recognizing cues, improving skill in listening, identifying cues and practising listening skills

Session 5
Reinforcing and encouraging
Verbal and non-verbal encouragements, praise, valuing, repeating and reflecting

Session 6
Information giving
The purpose of giving information, facilitating and inhibiting the effective passage of information factors related to each

Session 7
Opening and closing
Restrictions, time and environment, successful and unsuccessful openings and closings, factors leading to success, feelings and behaviour, review to date

Session 8
Comfort and reassurance
Patient-centred behaviour, nurse-centred behaviour, purpose, benefit, relationship formation, constructing barriers, research, health education, risk-taking, self-disclosure

(cont.)

Figure 11.1 Programme for micro skills in *CINE* project: the content of the 15 sessions (Faulkner and Macleod Clark, 1987).

Session 9
Combining micro skills
Nursing process: Assessing patients' and relatives' needs for communication, appropriate nursing behaviours, admission of a patient, problem identification, goals

Session 10
Communicating with other members of the health care team
Authority, power and control, roles, attitudes, organizations, accountability, assertion, advocacy

Session 11
Cancer and dying
Diagnosis, defensiveness, denial, detachment, death, dying process, trust, empathy, sharing, identification, self-awareness

Session 12
Preparing a patient for discharge
Health promotion, the nurse as a teacher, patients' rights, nurses' rights, education aims, alcoholism, heart disease, antenatal care, stoma patient discharge, smoking

Session 13
Communicating with and nursing geriatric and stroke patients
Defining inhibiting factors, physiological failure of sight, hearing, smell, taste, touch; movement, frustration, denial, anger, rejection

Session 14
Communicating with patients before and after surgery
Pre- and post-operative care, research findings, identifying fear, anxiety and recovery rate, reducing anxiety

Session 15
Investigations of surgical and medical patients
Verbal and non-verbal skills and strategies providing a framework for effective communication with patients and colleagues, encouraging effective communication with 'difficult', 'anxious' and 'depressed' patients

Figure 11.1 (*cont.*) Programme for micro skills in *CINE* project: the content of the 15 sessions (Faulkner and Macleod Clark, 1987).

difference between what is social interaction and what is professional interaction. Identifying differences between the two can help learners to realize that professional interaction is an art that has to be learnt (Faulkner, 1988).

In the CINE programme the link between micro skills and nursing was made by using transcripts of nurse/patient interaction and video demonstrations of nurse/patient interaction to illustrate the use of the particular skill being taught in any one session. Later, sessions that were built into a particular specialty, for example, surgery, would be linked to interacting with surgical patients and the skills that had been taught as micro skills would be consolidated by these links.

Further consolidation was achieved by asking nurses in the study to make tape-recordings of interactions with their patients. These tape-recordings were then transcribed and feedback given to students during classroom sessions (Chapter 5). The results of the CINE experience suggested that the exercise, which was treated as a joke by some people but taken very seriously by others, should be changed to encourage students to make recordings of their interviews during clinical allocation. The students would then be asked to do their own transcribing and analysis of the tapes to develop insight into their own performance and begin to make their own assessments, and from this they could themselves identify areas of need for further work and feedback.

THE BENEFITS OF MICRO SKILLS TEACHING

There are many benefits to teaching the use of a micro skills approach. Three major benefits will be described here.

1. By concentrating teaching on the actual skills to be learnt, participants are able to identify each particular skill and its components. For example, in the CINE project an hour was devoted to questioning techniques. During this time the students not only discussed the three main types of questions, that is, open, closed and leading, but also looked at the effects of using each type. They then considered the need to use a particular sort of question in detail and the factors controlling that decision. Also within the hour the students had the opportunity to work on transcribed conversations in terms of improving the dialogue through the skilful use of questioning technique.
2. The use of a micro skills approach allows each skill to be learned independently from the others. For example, most individuals would accept that if you want to hear what somebody is saying, you need to listen. In the CINE project an hour was spent on teaching the students about listening as a skilled activity. Time was given for practising listening and attending behaviours and assessing their own skills of listening effectively. Techniques of active listening were underlined with the aim of improving skills and heightening hearing awareness. If a session such as this is taught in a sensitive and interesting way it is unlikely that any student in the class will not realize that listening is

a complex skill that needs to be mastered. This holds true for all micro skills in the programme.

3. A third major advantage to the micro skills approach is that each skill is mastered before students are asked to link those skills with effective interaction with their patients. For example, Session 11 in the CINE programme concentrated on linking micro skills in the area of cancer and dying by using vignettes, role play and video demonstration. From this the students are able to identify, from their in-depth knowledge of micro skills (1) the exact skills that are being used, (2) how those skills work towards improved interaction, and (3) how the micro skills link together in effective dialogue.

THE DISADVANTAGES OF A MICRO SKILLS APPROACH

Although teaching micro skills can be very effective, there are disadvantages to this approach.

1. Sessions which concentrate on one skill at a time are often not taken seriously, particularly if non-contextualized exercises are used to underpin a concept. In the first (unpublished) workshops, where exercises were used to help individuals to consider the skills of communication, participants often complained that they did not seem to be much more than a party game. For example, in helping someone to understand the value of listening, exercises were used to show how important it is that other non-verbal behaviour is appropriate. This might mean, for example, trying to talk to someone back-to-back, to show that it is very difficult to listen when you are not looking at the person concerned. This would inevitably end with (1) some giggles, and (2) a certain amount of resentment arising from the belief that the participants were being treated like children. This problem of not taking micro skills teaching seriously does tend to fade once the skills are linked with the particular areas of concern that the student is covering. At this point, micro skills will begin to make sense.

2. From the above it can be seen that teaching micro skills independently from the context in which they are to be used can cause problems. The learners will not automatically see the relevance to clinical reality, especially in the early days of training to be a health professional when there is not a lot of clinical practice to underline the teaching. This problem was overcome to a certain extent in the CINE project by using transcripts and demonstration video tapes, but if the transcript was not related to the area that a nurse was particularly concerned with at the time, it was again not seen to be very relevant to the business of learning to become a nurse.

3. A major disadvantage to teaching micro skills is the limits on available time. If it is going to take an hour to teach each skill and

many more hours to integrate those skills into the context of health care, then considerable time needs to be devoted to the programme. It was interesting in the CINE project to find that 15 sessions were negotiated for the pilot study, but that this was reduced to 10 to 12 sessions in the main study. A further constraint is the time lag between each session. If, for example, micro skills are being taught one by one, then the sessions need to follow fairly closely on each other. If this does not happen then the student is left with a number of fragmented sessions that are quite difficult to put together when top-up sessions occur in different specialties. The skills that should be linked to particular areas of patient care may well need considerable revision. It is probably true to say that micro skills teaching is much more relevant to the basic nurse training or medical training programmes than it is to a workshop for qualified professionals, where participants could get very bored with studying one skill at a time. Context and time potential is very important when planning a particular approach.

TEACHING STRATEGIES

The Maguire/Faulkner model (1988) teaches strategies and skills required to enhance effective interaction in health care, with a major emphasis on assessment and the identification of patients' problems. This approach is particularly useful for multidisciplinary groups of trained staff, for it can build on existing skills and improve the participant's repertoire.

It was soon discovered that it cannot be assumed that participants will all have the skills required to communicate effectively, and they may not have had formal sessions on the skills required. This model concentrates on the skills required to elicit concerns and feelings from a psychosocial perspective. The strategies taught also include handling emotional situations such as anger, guilt and emotionally loaded situations. A typical programme for a workshop based on the Maguire/Faulkner (1988) model is shown in Figure 1.1.

Advantages of the model

The three main advantages of the model are as follows:

1. The teaching is tied tightly to the participant's clinical reality and no assumptions are made about what is relevant to a particular group. Obviously some sessions will be more relevant to some participants than others, but it is usually possible to get a balance so that participants all feel that their major concerns have been addressed. By

linking the teaching to clinical reality it also gives participants something to take away in terms of different approaches to problems in the future. This often has a knock-on effect in terms of what participants report when they return for follow-up days.

2. Another real advantage of the model is that the teaching methods demonstrate the approach to patient care that will be taught throughout the workshop or course. For example, when identifying the problem areas that participants want to cover in the workshop, it is pointed out that there are parallels between patients identifying their concerns, and participants on a course identifying the problem areas that they would like to address. It is then possible to draw further parallels in terms of what is possible in the workshop in that when a patient identifies their concerns, it is important to get some priority rating on those concerns since they cannot all be covered in one session. Similarly with the actual teaching, it is pointed out that priorities have to be given to the problem areas (see Chapter 12). By drawing attention to these parallels the model of care is reinforced throughout the course.

3. A third major advantage of the Maguire/Faulkner approach is that the participants feel totally involved in what is taught, in that the teaching is based on an agenda identified by them. This setting of an agenda invariably results in total commitment to what is taught so that the problems of motivation seldom arise. Further, the participants feel valued and trusted to identify their own needs.

Disadvantages of the model

There are disadvantages to the methods of teaching employed by Faulkner and Maguire, particularly given that much of the teaching concerns psychosocial aspects of care. There are three major disadvantages to the model.

1. Unless handled very carefully, there is a risk that participants will get to feel de-skilled at the beginning of the workshop when the model of care is demonstrated. It could be argued that this could also be true in the micro skills approach, in that many youngsters coming into nursing would feel it quite insulting to be taught to listen, to be taught how to question effectively, or to be taught other elements of communication. What makes a difference in the Maguire/Faulkner (1988) approach, is that all the teaching links to clinical reality so that the participant begins to think of the way they have operated prior to the workshop, and may begin to wonder if they have been 'doing it wrong' for many years. This problem needs to be identified and can be avoided by the positive approach to all feedback sessions.

2. There is a risk of triggering in any teaching that addresses psycho-social and emotional issues (see Chapter 7). Although this is not a common occurrence in workshops it is a potential problem, particularly since many individuals are unaware of the personal 'luggage' that they carry around in terms of unresolved problems or reactions to losses of various degrees of importance. This risk can be reduced by erring on the side of caution and safety in teaching, but for any teacher of communication skills who links their teaching to clinical reality, there is the need to develop the skills of screening the group and picking up problems sooner rather than later.

3. A third problem in the teaching of communication to participants who come from a variety of backgrounds and institutions is that at the end of the course that person may not be seen again by the course tutors. This puts constraints on the tutors that are very different from those of teaching people throughout a course of study, such as a degree, or a nurse training programme, where regular updates can be given. The problem of short workshops and the need to follow-up may be overcome by building in follow-up days some months after the first workshop. This is obviously appreciated by participants since in Help the Hospices workshops many of these participants have been back a third time to develop their ability to teach communication skills.

It can be seen from the above that there are advantages and disadvantages of teaching using the micro skills approach and using the strategy-plus-skills-based approach to teaching communication skills. It is argued here that micro skills teaching in the basic education of nurses and doctors would make a good foundation on which to base further teaching and development of skills using the approach where skills are incorporated into strategies to deal with the many interactive issues that arise for patients and their families when dealing with illness. In the CINE experience it was found that micro skills are best taught, absorbed and appreciated after the participant has had some clinical experience.

SUMMARY

In this chapter the skills of communication have been considered in terms of two methods of teaching. First, the micro skills approach as used in the CINE programme has been explored, along with the pros and cons of the method. Second, the Maguire/Faulkner (1988) approach has been considered in terms of clinically oriented teaching, which gives participants both the skills and strategies required to interact effectively with patients and their families. These two methods have been seen to be complementary rather than mutually exclusive since participants having a grounding in micro skills can then move on more readily to the clinically oriented approach and build on their skills in clinical practice.

REFERENCES

Faulkner, A. (1988) Effective communication. *Senior Nurse*, **8**(3), 5–6.

Faulkner, A. and Macleod Clark, J. (1987) Communication skills teaching in nurse education, in *Nursing Education: Research and Developments* (ed. B. Davis), Croom Helm, London.

Maguire, P. and Faulkner, A. (1988) How to improve counselling skills of doctors and nurses in cancer care. *British Medical Journal*, **297**, 847–9.

CHAPTER TWELVE

A model for teaching

TEACHING IN CONTEXT

When trained nurses, doctors and other health professionals come to workshops or seminars on effective interaction, they generally come because they are aware of some of their own deficiencies and are motivated to improve their skills. However, much teaching is concerned with students – student nurses, medical students and other undergraduates and students in health care. One of the biggest problems with student groups is in helping them to understand that there are things that they have to learn to improve their ability to communicate effectively with patients and their relatives and friends. Yet research has shown over and over again that the skills used in social interaction do not help nurses and other health professionals to interact effectively with patients (for example, Faulkner, 1985, 1992a).

Social versus professional interaction

In the CINE project (Chapter 10) it was found that student nurses saw little point in lectures on how to communicate with patients. Many of them argued that their ability to 'get on' with people was what led them into nursing. It was only when the nurses had experience of working with patients on the ward that they realized that there was something subtly different between talking to people in a social way and talking to people professionally when they or their loved ones were ill and needing care. This led to the belief that rather than teach micro skills as the whole of a programme on effective interaction, it was preferable to teach communication skills in the context of the participant's or student's own clinical reality. This means that in the undergraduate or student nursing programme, communication skills teaching should be deferred until after the first ward experience, and then introduced in terms of 'What sort of interactions did you have with patients and what were the problems?' As one student succinctly put it, 'I knew her diagnosis all right, but I wasn't sure why she'd asked me about it or how much I could tell her, or how, given that the news wasn't good.'

By eliciting problems that participants have experienced in their own clinical setting, it is possible to compare the model of interaction being taught (Faulkner, 1992b) with the method of teaching. This linking can remind students at a very early stage in their learning, first, that they can make no assumptions about what the problems are in the same way that the teacher is making no assumptions on what concerns the students and, second, that problems need to be identified before action is taken in the same way that the teacher is identifying the students' problems before getting into the 'meat' of the session on interaction.

This approach will work even if the bare bones of the programme have been planned before the course starts. For example, there may be a first session on assessment and the tutor can have prepared the material for that but by basing the general issues on problems identified by the student, a sense of reality is immediately brought into the learning. Similarly with other subjects that can be planned as outlines, with the students providing the problem-oriented material for discussion or role play or other teaching methods which may be used.

Developing an agenda

If, as in workshops (Maguire and Faulkner 1988), the majority of material is to be based on the participants' problems, then an agenda will need to be set prior to any major teaching input. This may seem a very risky way to approach teaching, but what is surprising is that the agenda generated by participants over many years of workshops has always included the majority of the material that the tutors wish to teach. If, however, there are areas that the tutors feel are vital to be taught, then they will negotiate with the participants in the same way that the health professional will negotiate with a patient when they need to screen in areas that have not been mentioned by that patient.

Setting an agenda

The following is a guide only to helping participants to set a realistic agenda on which future teaching will be based. First, the tutor will need to negotiate with the group that they themselves are the experts on what they need in order to improve their ability to communicate effectively with the patients and their families. The tutor might say something as follows:

'Although we have been running workshops like this for a considerable amount of time, one of the lessons that we've learned is that we cannot assume that we know precisely which areas are of most concern to any one group. Obviously there are issues which we, as your tutors, will want to raise in the same way that there are vital issues that you wish to raise with your patients, but as we hope you base your assessment of patients on the problems that they identify, we are going to base this workshop on problems that you identify. For this we think you should be working in small groups and we will later on divide you into two groups (of eight to ten).'

BRIEFING

It is important to spell out the task of the group precisely, for example:

'What we want you to do is to think of your own clinical experience over the last two to three months and to think of times when you came away from a situation feeling that somehow you could have handled it better. We hope you'll have time to share the good things, too, but what we need from you at the end of the exercise is three lists:

1. one of problem areas between yourselves and patients;
2. one of problem areas between yourselves and relatives, and;
3. one of problems between yourselves and colleagues.

'What you need to do is to get someone in the group to volunteer to report back, and we'd like a verbal report because then we can put it up on the flip chart in context. You also need to appoint someone in the group who will make sure that everybody gets a fair say because in any group, no matter how small, there's always somebody who will, if left to their own devices, do most of the talking, and at the other end of the scale there's often somebody who may not say anything even though they have agenda items.'

'For this exercise we want you to be very selfish, that is, if you have a problem, even if nobody else seems to have that problem, stay with it because what we want is that the workshop is important to you, and very often you'll find that your problem isn't isolated but is shared in some form or another by colleagues either in your own group or in the other group.'

'When you come back we'll get your lists from both groups up on the board and you'll see again a parallel between our teaching and your work, because when you identify your patients' problems it's very unusual that you deal with them all at once and I suspect that that's how it's going to be with us.'

'What is important is that you share *specific* rather than general problems. For this you will need to describe actual incidents – though of course you do not need to use the patient's name.'

'It's unlikely that you'll bring just enough problems to cover the time we've got together, so what we'll be asking you to do when we come back is to give some priority to the problems identified and again you will make that decision, not us, only rather than making it on a personal basis you'll make it as a consensus within the group.'

'Is everybody happy with the task? OK. Well, now we're going to split you into two groups and because it's important that you work with people that you don't know, because part of this exercise is getting to know each other, we'll label you 1, 2 ... around the room and then if you are sitting by a friend, that friend will be in another group. Sorry if that sounds mean.'

This exercise usually takes about an hour. That may seem quite a long time but part of the process is that individuals within the group begin to get to know each other.

If, for example, the workshop is followed up later on by another two days or so, then the time for agenda setting can be much reduced because the group members already know each other, but for a group meeting for the first time an hour gives them time to begin to memorize names and talk a bit about what they do. This starts the process of trust-building which makes it easier for individuals to bring up the problems that they wish to be addressed during the workshop.

The tutor or facilitator generally leaves the groups to work alone because then they are working as a peer group. This is a matter of personal choice, but at this early stage in a workshop the tutor can have an inhibiting effect on group members.

IDENTIFYING PRIORITIES

When the group reforms, the reporter from the first group is asked to list the problems identified by group members. There is a risk here that group members will have given very general problems unless they have been clearly briefed. For example, 'How do you really find out what's worrying patients?' The tutor then asks, 'Whose problem was this and can you tell me why you were particularly worried about it?' In this way the agenda items become much more focused than generalized and make later planning of the workshop easier. For example, if one were going to do a role play on assessment, it is much easier to take a scenario that has already been given by a participant than to think of one at the time from a general statement.

By making the agenda items specific to particular patients and situations, the skills of precision and clarification are underlined. Also, the particular student is encouraged to think clearly of the exact nature of the problem. When the reporter from group 1 has completed the list, the tutor then asks group 1 if anyone within the group has items that they feel have been omitted or which they have thought of since. The leader from group 2 is then asked to identify areas of overlap, of which there are often quite a few, but also to add items that were raised in that group which had not been raised in group 1. This then gives a reasonably complete picture of the whole group's problems and can generate perhaps more than 20 problem areas. Figure 1.2 (p. 13) shows a typical agenda for a multidisciplinary workshop for doctors, nurses and other health professionals.

Collating agenda items

The task for the tutor is then to organize the problems into a useable list that can be prioritized by the participants. For example, some of the problems can go together as part of the same area. It may be that one of the problems is identifying patients' real concerns. Another may be time management. Yet another may be helping a patient to express himself. These three could all go under the general area of assessment, which will include organizing time, identifying problems and helping a patient to disclose fears, worries and feelings. When setting priorities it is important that participants are aware of the context of each area identified.

The priority list

One method of prioritizing (Maguire and Faulkner, 1988) is to give the participants 10 points for every problem listed. It is explained that 10 is the maximum score for a problem that is of vital importance to the participant and that nought is the minimum score for an area either of no concern, not applicable, or because the individual participant feels that they are already competent in that area. Participants are alerted to the fact that they can easily be led into giving a score that is not appropriate to them. For example, if several people in a row give a score of eight, it is a big temptation for the next participant to also say eight, so again participants are asked to be quite selfish in their scoring and not to be afraid to give everything either a high score or a low score.

There is some room for humour here in terms of everything having a low score, the tutor might say, 'You can give everything nought if that's how you feel about it, but we will then give you the time of the next train home.' In other words, what usually happens is that each participant will give a range of scores from quite low in some areas to very high in others.

In putting together those problems that fit under one heading, for example, assessment, the eventual problem list will be around 15 to 18. When all the scores have been given, the tutor will offer to add the scores and put up the participants' top 10 problems. It is pointed out that this again parallels patient care in that when a patient has many problems, the ones that are worked with are those that are perceived, by the patient, as being most important and that others are given some attention at a later date or at a different level from the others. The participants are promised that before the end of the programme there will be a session on 'unfinished business' and that this session will include any of the top 10 items that have not been covered, though this is rare, and also the other problems that were given priority by the participants but nevertheless were not in the top ten.

Tutor's agenda

The tutors at some point in this negotiation should make quite clear what their own agenda items are. These would normally include: (1) the skills of basic assessment; and (2) support and survival.

The rationale for this is the belief that accurate assessment of current problems is central to planning effective patient care and that the professional's own welfare is paramount if good care is to be delivered. If these arrive in the top 10 of the participants' agenda, obviously the whole workshop is based on that agenda, but if they are low scoring or not in the agenda at all, then the tutor needs to clarify why they are going to add these agenda items. It will need to be explained that assessment is seen as the basis for all interaction and therefore is a basic brick that cannot be omitted without risking the whole of the workshop misfiring. Second, the area of support and survival is seen to be vital because if the carers do not care for themselves, then they will not survive to go on doing their work. This is an area where participants often do not perceive or admit to problems partly because of their work ethic which may be based on a belief that the patients come first no matter what, but also because they feel that somehow they are expected to cope. Finding that they cannot always cope, nor yet should they be expected to do so, can be quite a momentous learning experience. One medical director of a hospice on completing a workshop run by Help the Hospices wrote in to say that the most useful thing in his personal life that he had gained from the workshop was the feeling that he had the right occasionally to say no.

THE PROGRAMME

Content

Following on the prioritizing of agenda items comes negotiation with the group on what is to be taught over the next few days. This is necessary because it may be believed by the participants that the highest scoring item will be dealt with first, where in fact the tutors have to look at the top 10 items and turn them into a cohesive programme that will start at a relatively safe level, moving on to more complex areas. It is usual to set the scene for the teaching to come by a 'chalk and talk' session on a common language of communication, followed by the basic skills of assessment, and from this the other material should fall neatly into place using the various methods used in earlier chapters of this book.

Finally, it is explained to the participants that what will be taught are skills and strategies. Hopefully, participants will find that these skills and strategies are generalizable to other situations, and this is one of the learning experiences that often happens over the course of the workshop. It is made clear that although these strategies have been found to work for the tutors, they are not written on tablets of stone and that rather than being in the business of producing clones, what tutors do want is to help participants to develop their own style and method of effective interaction with patients and their families, and to build on the strengths that they have brought with them, rather than being made to feel deskilled and having the resultant worry about past clinical practice.

Methods

The variety of methods to be used should be negotiated with participants with emphasis on the move from safe to less safe, and on the value of group participation the tutor may say:

> 'We shall use a variety of teaching methods to cover your agenda, with a minimum of chalk and talk, for we hope for considerable input from you. Some areas will be covered by video demonstration, where you will have the opportunity to constructively critique interactions, some sessions will rely on group discussion, and then we will move on to sessions where you will have a chance to practise in a relatively safe environment. Before we start has anyone questions that they wish to ask?'

A number of questions usually follows which gives the tutor an opportunity to explain, negotiate and reassure if this is appropriate. The tutor can then move on to the expected level of participation:

For a multidisciplinary group of doctors, nurses, social workers and others.

> 'We recognize that there is a considerable amount of expertise in this room although all/most/some of you have told us that you are here to improve skills. What we hope to do is to build on those skills but also to share your expertise. This means that we will be asking you to participate in video critique, in discussion and in generating ideas and solutions. Are you happy with that?'

For student nurses, medical students and other untrained staff.

> 'Although you are all learners you have already had a chance to work with/observe/interact with patients and their families. We hope that

you will feel able to share your ideas and experiences with the group and that you will also learn by testing those ideas and theories in a relatively safe environment.'

Most learners work well in an environment that encourages them to think through issues once the basic theory of effective interaction has been covered.

This approach respects that which each individual brings to the course, maintains interest and encourages motivation. Research (Faulkner, 1992a) suggests that participants improve skills rapidly.

SUMMARY

In this chapter it has been argued that a group will be more motivated to improve interactive skills if the teaching is linked with the participants' own clinical reality and the problems that they face in their day-to-day work. It has also been suggested that teaching is based either partially or wholly on an agenda identified by the members of the group which is then focused into distinct areas based on particular problems with patients, relatives or colleagues.

The whole group decides which of these areas are of greatest priority and the teaching is based on a consensus of concerns that are given in-depth treatment, and then the group is reassured that other areas which have been identified but which have not been given top priority will be headlined as unfinished business. If basic assessment and support and survival of the carers are not in the top 10, then the tutors will give those areas priority for reasons which they will negotiate with the group.

Teaching is then based on skills and strategies for the particular situations identified by the group and the generalizability of these skills and strategies to other areas of care.

REFERENCES

Faulkner, A. (1985) Evaluation of teaching interpersonal skills in nursing, in *Communication* (ed. C. Kagan), Croom Helm, London.

Faulkner, A. (1992a) The evaluation of training programmes for communication skills in palliative care. *Journal of Cancer Care*, **1**(2), 75–8.

Faulkner, A. (1992b) *Effective Interaction with Patients*, Churchill Livingstone, Edinburgh.

Maguire, P. and Faulkner, A. (1988) How to improve the counselling skills of doctors and nurses in cancer care. *British Medical Journal*, **297**, 847–9.

Appendix: Resources

FURTHER READING

Argyle M. (1983) *The Psychology of Interpersonal Behaviour*, 4th edn, Penguin, Harmondsworth.

Bond, M. (1986) *Stress and Self-Awareness: A Guide for Nurses*, Heinemann Nursing, London.

Bridge, W. and Macleod Clark, J (eds) (1981) *Communication in Nursing Care*, HM & M Publishers, London.

Buckman, R. (1990) *I Don't Know What to Say: How to Help and Support Someone Who is Dying*, Rev. ed. Papermac, London.

Burnard, P. (1989) *Counselling Skills for Health Professions*, Chapman & Hall, London.

Corny, R. (ed) (1991) *Developing Communications and Counselling Skills in Medicine*, Routledge, London.

Davis, B. and Ternulf-Nhylin, K. (1982) *The Assessment of Training in Social Skills in Nursing, With Particular Reference to the Patient Profile Interview. Issues in Nursing Research*, Macmillan Press Ltd., London, 121–33.

Fallowfield, L. (1990) *The Quality of Life: The Missing Measurement in Health Care*, Souvenir Press, London.

Faulkner, A. (1992) *Effective Interaction with Patients*, Churchill Livingstone, Edinburgh.

Faulkner, A. (1992) Communication skills in cancer and palliative care: the need to evaluate. *Medical Encounter*, **8**(4), 8–10.

Faulkner, A., Maguire, P. and Regnard, C. (1993) The angry patient or relative. *Palliative Medicine* (in press).

Faulkner, A., Webb, P. and Maguire, P. (1991) Communication and counselling skills: educating health professionals working in cancer and palliative care. *Patient Education and Counselling*, **18**, 3–7.

Jackson, E. (1989) *Understanding Health: An Introduction to the Holistic Approach*, SCM Press, London.

Kagan, C. (1985) *Interpersonal Skills in Nursing*, Croom Helm, London.

Kagan, C. (1987) *A Manual of Interpersonal Skills for Nurses*, Harper & Row, London.

Knox, J.D.E. and Thompson, G.M. (1989) Breaking bad news: medical undergraduate communication skills teaching and learning. *Medical Education*, **23**, 258–61.

Krieger, D. (1979) *The Therapeutic Touch*, Prentice Hall, Englewood Cliffs, New Jersey.

Maguire, P. (1988) The stress of communicating with seriously ill patients. *Nursing*, **3**(32), 25–7.

Maguire, P., Faulkner, A. and Regnard, C. (1993) Eliciting the current problems of the patient with cancer. Flow diagram. *Medicine*, **7**, 63–8.

Maguire, P., Faulkner, A. and Regnard, C. (1993) Managing the anxious patient with advancing disease: A flow diagram. *Palliative Medicine*, **7**, 239–44.

Maguire, P., Faulkner, A. and Regnard, C. (1993) The Withdrawn Patient. *Palliative Medicine* (in press).

Marson, S. (1990) *Managing People*, Macmillan, London.

Pearson, A. (ed) (1987) *Nursing Quality Measurement*, John Wiley, Chichester.

Price, B. (1990) *Body Image: Nursing Concepts and Care*, Prentice Hall, Englewood Cliffs, New Jersey.

Robinson, E.J. and Whitfield, M.J. (1988) Contributions of patients to general practitioners' consultations in relation to their understanding of doctors' instructions and advice. *Social Science and Medicine*, **27**(9), 895–900.

Sale, D. (1990) *Quality Assurance*, Macmillan, London.

Vachon, M. (1987) *Occupational Stress in the Care of the Critically Ill, the Dying and the Bereaved*, Hemisphere, London.

Verby, J. *et al.* (1979) Peer reviews of consultations in primary care: the use of audiovisual recordings. *British Medical Journal*, **1**, 1686–8.

VIDEO–TAPES

The following video-tapes are useful for teaching purposes. Although developed for those working in cancer and terminal care, the skills and strategies are transferable to general health care.

Pfizer Drug Company (1992) Three 12-minute video-tapes on breaking bad news, each complete in itself (free on request from Pfizer).

1. *Breaking Bad News to a Patient.*
2. *Breaking Bad News to Relatives.*
3. *Breaking Bad News to Parents.*

Help the Hospices (1985) Five video-tapes with teaching notes.

1. *Basic Assessment.*
2. *The Difficult Patient.*
3. *The Young Angry Patient.*
4. *Collusion.*
5. *Advocacy.*

Help the Hospices tapes are £30 each in VHS format, £33 each in North American format and are available from Professor Ann Faulkner, Sykes House, Little Common Lane, Abbey Lane, Sheffield. Cheques made payable to 'Education account'.

Screne Productions Ltd (1991) *Child of a Dying Parent*. This video was sponsored by Help the Hospices and comes complete with teaching notes.

Screne Productions tape costs £50; also available from Professor Ann Faulkner. Cheques made payable to Help the Hospices (Trading) Ltd.

Index

Page numbers appearing in **bold** refer to figures.

Agenda
  collating items   130
  developing   127–8
  setting   127–8
  tutor's   131
Audio feedback   49–62
  audio-tape use   54–5, 102
  briefing notes   **51**
  conclusion   57–8
  feedback session   55–7
  interviews in clinical setting   50
  interviews with simulated patients
    50–52
  introduction to participants   52–4
  planning   49–52
  potential difficulties (audio-taped
    interviews)   58–61
    no suitable patient   58–9
    no time   60
    too nervous   60–61
    unsuitable interviewee   59–60
  schedule   **53**
Audio-tape   18, 54–5

Briefing   128–9
Burn out   90

Cancer Research Campaign,
    community nurse teaching   111
Captive audience   9
Cascade Project   113–14
Common language   18–19
  identification   17–18
  objectives   18–19
  session   19–22
  time allotment   19
Communication in Nurse Education
    (CINE)   109, 110–11
  preparation for teachers   111
  see also micro skills

Communication skills   117–25
  workshop generated   **20**
Competition element   17
Coping mechanisms   89, 92
Cost of caring, handling   88–96
Counselling   16
  skills   16

Discussion session   63–73
  full group with facilitator   72
  planning session   64–6
  potential problems   71–2
  sculpting   67–71
    changing positions   **69**
  session   66–8
  small group with no facilitator
    72–3
  subject choice   63–4
Disruptive participant   83–5
Distance-learning   106
Distress   94–5

Effective interaction strategies
    teaching   109–15
Evaluation   97–106
  formal   101–4
  global feedback from audio-tape
    102
  informal   97
  measuring effects over time   105
  open   97–9
  tick list form   100–101
  written   99–101, **103**, **104**
Exercises   7

Ground rules   93–4
Group   5–7
  captive audience   9
  cohesion   7
  expertise within   15–16

Group (*cont.*):
  introductions   10–11
  self-selection   9
  size   6–7
  working within   9

Health Education Council   109
Help the Hospices workshops   6, 63,
    113, 114
Hostile group   86–7

Late arriver   85–6
Learning from research   14–15

Maguire/Faulkner teaching model
    12, 122–4
  advantages   122–3
  disadvantages   123–4
Method selection   11–12
Micro skills   117–22
  benefits   120–21
  disadvantages   121–2
  teaching   117–20

Non-participator   81–2

Over-participator   82–3

Parameter setting   16–17
Participation negotiation   17–18
Personal vs professional issues   77–9
Planning   88–90
Potential difficulties (problems)
    77–87, 94–5
  disruptive participant   83–5
  hostile group   86–7
  late arriver   85–6
  non-participator   81–2
  over-participator   82–3
  personal vs professional issues
      77–9
  triggering   79–81
Priorities identification   129–30
Priority list   130–31
Professional support   93
Programme   131–3
  content   131–2
  method   132–3
  planning   11–13

Relevant tasks   7–9
Role play   34–48
  alibis   46
  briefing   40–44

  "patient"   41–2
  professional   42–3
  reality base   41–2
  chairs grouping   **40**
  concluding   47–8
  contracting   38
  differing views   46–7
  effect on group   47
  focus   38–9, 45–7
  making task explicit   36
  no personal experience   35
  positive feedback   34
  responsibility   36
  role   35
  role player effect   46
  safety rules   **37**
  size of group   36–7
  stop points   44–5
    player in difficulties   45
    teaching points   45
    time out   34–5, 44
  time   37
  volunteers gaining   39–40
    heirarchy of difficulty   39
    value of experience   39–40
  unsuitable areas   38–9

Scene setting   15
Session   90–94
  concluding   94
Simulator   50
Social vs professional interaction   126
Student
  demands on   4–5
  participation   4–5
  reactions   4
  safety feelings   5
  threat of experiential methods   5
Student set agenda   3
Support   89–90
Surveys, national
  directors of nurse education   109–10
  nurse tutors   109–10

Teaching model   126–33
Tension easing   17
Timing   90
Trent Palliative Care Centre   105
Triggering 79–81
Tutor
  demands on   3–4
    finding positives   4
  national survey   109–10
  responsibility   5–9

Value on self 88–92
Video-taped material 23–33
  large group 27–8
  potential problems 28–31
  session 25–7
    notes 25
    planning 24–5

stopping points 26–7
small group 28
value of producing material 31–2

Workshops 112–13
  Help the Hospices 6, 63, 113, 114